HEALTHY WEALTHY & WISE

KRS EDSTROM

WITH STEPHANIE NELSON
Foreword by Russ Hanlin, CEO, Sunkist Growers, Inc.

SOFT
STONE
Los Angeles, California

Formerly published in hardcover by:
Prentice Hall, 1993 ISBN: 0-13-296906-8
K. Edstrom ISBN: 1-886198-75-6

Library of Congress Cataloging Card Number: 98-94028

ISBN   1-886198-76-4

Cover Photo Credit: Glenn Vinzant

soft
STONE   Soft Stone Publishing
Post Office Box 8584
Los Angeles, California 91618-8584

Printed in the United States of America

ABOUT THE AUTHOR

KRS Edstrom, M.S., is a lecturer and advice columnist whose work has been featured in *USA Today, Wall Street Journal, Los Angeles Times, Glamour, Chicago Tribune, First For Women, Entrepreneur, Fitness* and *Kiplinger's Personal Finance Magazine*. Her guided meditation audios have been used as in-flight relaxation programming by US Airways, American and United Airlines. Hospitals, psychologists and many other practitioners use KRS' products. Her advice column, "Ask KRS," appears, among other places, in *Elle* and *Mirabella* magazines on American Online.

KRS conducts transformational HealthStyle Retreats, combining information with experience in peaceful settings. Her technique blends external and internal modalities—practical skills together with meditation, imagery and energy work. Her approach has been implemented in a variety of life challenges, including stress, pain, weight management, smoking, illness and even the dying process. Participants learn to turn inward, becoming self-educated and more responsible for every aspect of their mental, physical and spiritual health. KRS uses her master's degree in Health Science, her study of academic and alternative health and more than 20 years of practical experience to help corporations and private clients reach their goals and improve the quality of their lives.

Also by KRS Edstrom*

Conquering Stress (book)
Time Out For Time In (booklet)
Relax Mind & Body (audio)
Defeat Pain (audio)
Conquer Stress (audio)
Sleep Through Insomnia (audio)
Everyday Meditation (audio)
Instrumentals I (audio)

* See last page for ordering information

To Mom and Dad

and those committed to freeing themselves
of their limitations—
with plenty of smiles and music
along the way.

THANKS

These people keep me laughing, thinking, and/or grounded, and I welcome this chance to let them know.

Mary Edstrom — buddy, adviser, provider of laughs, love, and life. My "constant."

Ev Edstrom — alias "Hal Leonard," a world-class teacher and student, who at times taught me more about motivation than I thought I wanted to learn. Thanks, Dad — it all came in handy.

Steve — a funny and talented brother who suggested my profession. I hope he wasn't kidding...

My sisters — Pat, supporter and creator of my two favorite little people; Kate, thoughtful, open ear; and Kim, who keeps the laughs coming relentlessly.

Shinzen Young — meditation/life teacher and personal guide to expanding inward.

Glenn Vinzant — patient, caring confidant who knows more about me (and this book) than a person should have to know.

My clients — friends and teachers courageous enough to explore new forks in the road.

Friends and supporters — Nancy Stearn, Syd Silverman, Cindi Anderson, Hugh Penton, Curt Matthews, Jeff Harrington, Shirley Koster, Terry & Teresa James, Debby Young, Bernie & Dawn at Michele Audio, David & Cheryl at McNaughton & Gunn, Billie Temple, the "Other" Edstroms, Catherine-The-Great, Teri, Bill, Paula, Bluebird and a bunny called Lassiter.

*SPECIAL THANKS TO MY HEALTHY, WEALTHY & WISE LEADERS**

"Rocky" Johnson
CEO, Chairman of the Board
GTE

Kay Koplovitz
CEO, President
USA Network

Malcolm Stamper
President
Boeing Company

Paul Oreffice
Chairman of the Board
Dow Chemical

Brian Dyson
President, CEO
Coca-Cola Enterprises

Paul Allaire
CEO, Chairman
Xerox

David Miller
President
J.C. Penney

William Howell
CEO, Chairman of the Board
J.C. Penney

Marcia Israel
CEO, President
Judy's

Eileen Ford
Chairman of the Board
Ford Models

Robert Wycoff
President
Atlantic Richfield Co.

Colombe Nicholas
President
Christian Dior

James Kinnear
CEO
Texaco

Paul Lego
CEO
Westinghouse

Robert Schaeberle
CEO
Nabisco

Peter Magowan
CEO, Chairman of the Board
Safeway Stores

---

* Titles and company affiliations are from time of interview. In the interest of maintaining the impact of the findings, many titles and affiliations have been maintained throughout the text although changes have since occurred.

Mary Kay Ash
Chairman
Mary Kay Cosmetics

Kathryn Klinger
President
Georgette Klinger

James Evans
Chairman of the Board
Union Oil

Lawrence DelSanto
CEO, Chairman
Lucky Stores

Allen Jacobson
CEO, Chairman of the Board
3M

Paula Kent Meehan
CEO, Chairman
Redken Laboratories

Dr. Robert Boni
CEO, Chairman
Armco, Inc.

Randy Barron
President
Southwestern Bell

Allan Belzer
President
Allied Signal

Bruce Smart, Jr.
CEO, President
Continental Group

Ben Fauber
CEO, Chairman of the Board
K-Mart

Richard Mahoney
CEO
Monsanto

James Sullivan
Vice Chairman
Chevron

Richard Morrow
CEO
Amoco Oil

Philip Smith
President
General Foods

Debbie Fields
CEO, President
Mrs. Fields' Cookies

These are a few of the exceptional and remarkably giving people who have helped make this book possible.

KRS Edstrom

FOREWORD

Russ Hanlin, CEO and President
Sunkist

Great ideas are usually uncomplicated. KRS Edstrom had one: simply interview America's corporate leadership about success and healthful living in search of revealing patterns.

She found them.

Despite stressful burdens of responsibility and heavy workloads, Captains of Industry are uncommonly healthy. Quite separately, they have developed identifiable similarities. No fanatics here. Instead, comfortable but sensible diet and exercise habits are accompanied by a positive outlook, humor, and a sense of self-worth that predated promotion to executive status. Through KRS Edstrom's perceptiveness, we see that health involves the whole person, not just the physical being.

This is a happy, fascinating study that provides practical guidance.

INTRODUCTION

WHAT THIS BOOK CAN DO FOR YOU

"This is more than a program. It is a way of thinking and living."

Healthy, Wealthy & Wise is for busy women and men who can't seem to make results last. It is a "life management" program that is uniquely designed to accommodate your life when you can't make taking care of yourself a full-time job. For example, it shows you how to fit exercise and stretches into your normal workday or how to lose weight if you're not willing to entirely forego sweets.

Statistics show that although 70% of us know what we *should* be doing to take better care of ourselves, most of us still are not *doing* those things. *Healthy, Wealthy & Wise* includes a complete Motivation Program that helps you troubleshoot failure and stay motivated to insure long-term results. You will learn how to out-motivate distractions and excuses with mental tactics such as Reprogramming, Self-Dialoguing, Habit Strategy and Exer-psychology.

First, you'll be inspired by the leaders in this book as they give you their personal formulas for keeping fit both physically and mentally. As one said, "Health *is* success...it's one of the ways you keep score." Next, you'll be given KRS' powerful Eleven Proven Steps to Motivation and an easy-to-follow, doable program that is based on your particular needs and personality. Single people and families will love the revolutionary Speed Cooking Plan. It is an A-B-C approach to shopping, cooking, menu planning and eating that makes preparing a meal for one or seven as convenient as picking up fast food.

This book will help you meet mental and physical challenges, reduce stress, manage your time and lose weight. You will evolve not only more fit in body, mind and spirit, but with more self-knowledge and a life of quality.

ABOUT THIS BOOK

Healthy, Wealthy & Wise grew out of an extensive study conducted by KRS Edstrom on the health habits of America's highest ranked corporate leaders. The results of the study point to one overwhelming conclusion: *Good health and success are intimately connected.* Significantly, the majority of the men and women KRS interviewed changed to more healthful lifestyles *before* they made it to the top, and a commitment to good health remains a major factor in maintaining their success today. As you will learn, "success" is not meant to be exclusively defined as running a major corporation. According to one leader, "Success is simply achieving what you set out to do."

Here is a profile of the average leader interviewed:

- Average age 55
- Became serious about health at 35
- Was financially successful at 39
- Weighs twelve pounds less than the average American by height
- Married 29 years (compared to 6½ years for the average American!)
- Exercises three times a week or more
- Has been exercising regularly for 18 years
- Travels on business 13½ weeks a year
- Received no financial support from parents

ABOUT THE STUDY

The study revealed in *Healthy, Wealthy & Wise* is unique in that it is *based on personal interviews*, unlike any other study of this nature. The corporations in the core study are an exclusive representation of the top 100 publicly owned companies in America, as ranked per highest sales volume by Dun and Bradstreet at the time of this study. An unprecedented 56 percent—more than half—of these target companies participated. Including KRS' second study of top-ranked women business leaders, 69 companies represented by 87 corporate leaders participated in this study. In the interest of maintaining the impact of the findings, many titles and affiliations have been maintained throughout the text although changes have since occurred.

FROM THE AUTHOR

In observing my mother and father overcome a lifetime of challenges worthy of a TV mini-series, I learned a lot about struggling, survival and success. It seems they just kept (and keep) getting up and figuring a way over, around or through. When I was handed my own customized package of obstacles, I took the long way around before recruiting those lessons. Helping others take "a shorter way around" eventually became my work.

Living in California, one is subject to abrupt reminders of how impermanent things really are. Each time I feel the earth move (in the literal sense) and find myself standing in a flimsy doorframe, fervently making new resolutions while feeling something between silly and terrified, I am forced to recall the ephemeral nature of this whole thing. My hope is that this book will help guide you in evolving the quality of your stay while appreciating life's assignments and excursions along the way.

"Good stuff! Puts diet and exercise in perspective. Losing weight and getting in shape is not going to work unless it's part of a person's normal routine and isn't a hassle. You just do it—you don't think about it. I can also personally recommend KRS' stress and pain management techniques. They work!"

– Augie Nieto, CEO, Lifecycle

"Provides a clear explanation of why diet, exercise and stress reduction improve health and productivity, as well as practical tips that keep you motivated in achieving your goals."

– Paul Rosch, M.D., President,
The American Institute of Stress

"A terrific must for anybody who wants to stay alive and protect his or her health."

– William P. Castelli, M.D., Director,
Framingham Heart Study

"If it is true that you can't argue with success, then it is also true you can't argue with this book—it tells you what success is made of. The only way it wouldn't change your life is if you're already following the principles it describes."

– Rudolph M. Ballentine, M.D., Author,
Diet & Nutrition: A Holistic Approach

"*Healthy, Wealthy & Wise* is a practical no excuses recipe for a healthy working lifestyle."

– Richard McKegney, General Manager,
National Bank of Kuwait, Singapore

CONTENTS

Part Two
TAKING ACTION
The HWW HealthStyle Program   107

Chapter Six / **Managing Your Time for Health and Success   117**

Chapter Seven / **A Better HealthStyle Starts in Your Head:
Mental Fitness Training   127**

Chapter Eight / **The Healthy, Wealthy & Wise Mental Fitness
Program   143**

Part One

GETTING MOTIVATED:

SUCCESSFUL
HEALTHSTYLE STRATEGIES

Most of us die with our music unplayed. We use only 10 percent of our God-given abilities. We should try to step out of our comfort zones and do the things we're capable of.

—Mary Kay Ash, Chairman, Mary Kay Cosmetics

1

Chapter One

*T*HE
*H*EALTH-*S*UCCESS
*C*ONNECTION

It's hard to separate health and success.
— *Richard Morrow, CB, CEO emeritus, Amoco Oil*

How do you define success? Is it fame, fortune or completing the Boston Marathon? Is it a successful relationship? Raising a family? Painting a masterpiece? How much of your definition is colored by how others define success? Clarifying this is vital because chasing "success" as defined by others is an uncatchable carrot that can cost you a lifetime of unhappiness.

The study I conducted on the heads of America's top corporations, including Coca-Cola, GTE and J.C. Penney, has revealed how these powerful men and women succeeded in reaching the pinnacle of happiness and success as defined by *them* and no one else.

I asked them detailed questions about their mental outlook, their jobs, their personal lives and their health practices. I found that these corporate giants are *self-made* and have achieved success through their own initiative. I would describe them not as ladder climbers but as masters at knowing themselves and taking care of themselves. Not coincidentally, they became successful in their endeavors. Their secrets, together with my Healthy, Wealthy & Wise HealthStyle Program, can now be your own most powerful resource in attaining personal and professional goals that will not only bring you happiness, but success as defined by *you*.

What is the bottom line for these men and women? *More than 93 percent agree that health and success are intimately connected, and the overwhelming majority practice what they preach.* As you will see, they shatter the long-standing image of successful people as self-sacrificing workaholics with stressful, cutthroat jobs, three-martini lunches, and minimal home lives.

While their workdays are busy and demanding, these leaders *make* time to stay fit, a priority that has gotten them to the top and helps keep them there. Dow Chemical's CEO, Paul Oreffice, admits: "It's easy to let your business schedule dictate your life, particularly in the beginning. There's always an excuse not to do your exercise, especially in the morning when you're in a hurry and rushing around. You absolutely *have* to make health part of your priority. Now, I would no more think of leaving the house in the morning without exercising than without getting dressed. It's just part of my life." It must be—at the time I interviewed him, Paul had not missed a single workout in eleven years!

Coca-Cola's Brian Dyson firmly believes that "It will soon be medically proven that if you are healthy, you have more confidence and peace of mind, handle pressure better, need less sleep, and have more acuity." Brian epitomizes the American dream. He left Argentina at age 23 to join Coca-Cola in Venezuela, and by age 43 was president of Coca-Cola USA. Maintaining 10.5 percent body fat, Brian is a triathlete who trains no less than an hour a day and faithfully keeps up his workouts during the twenty weeks a year that he travels.

Brian Dyson comes close to being religious about the benefits of healthy living. And his convictions are echoed by the others whose lives are examined in this book. They recognized the value of getting and staying healthy, and have reaped the rewards.

Along with giving them the stamina to make it to the top, better diet and exercise pay off in many other ways for these high-ranking men and women. This can be measured by the ultimate yardstick—the fact that they live longer. According to one study, upper management, white-collar workers in America live four years longer, on average, than their peers.

Besides living longer, they are also closer to their ideal weights than their American peers and have healthier vital statistics as well. The average male I interviewed has a serum cholesterol level of 201, compared with 237 for the average American male in his age group. And his blood pressure is 127/83, compared with 134/87 for his American peers.

If having "good numbers" doesn't impress you, feeling good and needing less sleep should certainly interest you. Paradoxically, these leaders have more energy than the rest of us but need less sleep (6.9 hours versus 7.5 hours per night).

The way most of us live is "hazardous to our health." By some estimates, 83 percent of American deaths under age 65 could be prevented. This is based on the fact that the top five causes of death in this country are considered lifestyle related, that is, *preventable.* Heart disease is the leading cause of death in men aged 35 to 54. In fact, an estimated 1.5 million Americans will have heart attacks this year, many of which could have been prevented through healthier living.

What can we learn from these statistics? If you are serious about achieving your goals, *plan what goes into your mouth and get those feet moving.* Being successful, however you define it, is a lot easier if you're in shape. Or as one CEO put it: "It's pretty hard to be successful if you're dead."

HOW AMERICA'S MOST SUCCESSFUL WOMEN BALANCE CAREER, FAMILY, AND HEALTH

The women who participated in my study are owners of, or key decision makers in, some of the top money-making businesses in the United States. They were selected from the Savvy 60, a roster of America's top money-making female business owners, and from *Business Week's* roster of the fifty highest-ranking women in corporate America.

Aside from success, what do these women have in common? And in what ways do they differ from their male peers? I found that the lives of these women are more hectic and demanding than the lives of their male counterparts. A quote from Mary Kay Ash, founder of Mary Kay Cosmetics, says it all: "I hit the floor running and race the clock all day." In addition to being business leaders, most are also homemakers, mothers, and wives. However, unlike the males, the females don't have the full-time support of wives.

As overloaded as they are, most of the women work health and fitness into their lives. The majority have health habits that are better than the average American and almost as good as those of the males I studied. "I put my workout on my daily calendar. I think anyone can do this at any level," says Kay Koplovitz, CEO and president of USA Network.

Significantly, the women I studied believe that a good HealthStyle helps give them the strength to battle their biggest enemy—pressure. "Anyone who has as much stress in their life as I do had better be healthy," warns Kathryn Klinger, president of Georgette Klinger.

Redken's CEO, Paula Kent Meehan, believes that good health promotes success, but also believes that success can bolster one's health: "I'm almost superstitious about it," she says. "You don't have time to worry about every little sore throat or whatever if you're busy and involved." Or, as Marcia Israel, founder of the chic Judy's clothing chain, puts it: "Success gives you health." Indeed, important research now shows that a healthy, happy emotional state directly and dramatically affects your immune system. The women in this book give further credibility to studies that say that women who function in multiple roles (i.e., career woman, mother, and wife) appear to be healthier than other women. One such study was conducted by epidemiologist Donna Kritz-Silverstein at the University of San Diego School of Medicine. Kritz-Silverstein studied women in high-ranking jobs and found them more likely to have a healthier lifestyle than women in lower-ranking jobs. They exercised more and drank and smoked less, which would contribute to their longevity. But, perhaps most importantly, these women *enjoyed* their work. In fact, Kritz-Silverstein believes that employment may be a factor in longevity only if the woman *enjoys what she does*.

How do the women in my study stack up against the men? The typical female is 8.5 years younger than her male counterpart, and her overall health practices are slightly less rigorous, particularly when it comes to exercise. Compared with her male peers who participated in this study, the typical female:

- Exercises one hour a week less than the males.
- Is more likely to skip breakfast or lunch.
- Works longer hours.
- Sleeps less.
- Travels more (15 weeks a year, versus 13.5 weeks a year for males).
- Takes more vitamins.
- Drinks even less alcohol and coffee than the male.

UP CLOSE AND PERSONAL: HEALTHSTYLE PROFILES OF NINE TOP AMERICAN LEADERS

On the following pages are HealthStyle profiles of nine busy but generous successes who participated in my study. You'll find their words and HealthStyles both enlightening and inspiring. What comes through most clearly is that these men and women are vital, energetic people who genuinely love life and aren't afraid of its challenges. They are truly in their prime, although many are in their sixties and even beyond (the average man is 55) and they are all true believers in the health-success connection.

KAY KOPLOVITZ
CEO, President
USA Network

Age: 40s

Weight: Normal. "Everybody always wants to lose five pounds."

Married?: Yes

Energy: "To be high energy, you have to be healthy. Eating less and exercising more keeps my energy level up."

Fitness Motivation: Kay has memories of obesity and ill health as a child. "Now I feel strong and healthy, and that motivates me—I want to stay that way."

Diet: Low salt, low sugar, low fat, doesn't smoke, doesn't drink daily. Eats no red meat. Has two cups of coffee a day.

Meals:
  Breakfast—hard roll, coffee or fruit and cereal, egg once a week.
  Lunch—fish, vegetable, fruit.
  Dinner—Her secret: No large dinners. She "grazes" on vegetables, fruit, grains.

Favorite Foods: Fish, vegetables, ice cream. "It's hard to beat a really good piece of fish or really good vegetables." She eats ice cream rarely now.

Vitamins: C, B complex, calcium.

Exercise: Low-impact aerobics and calisthenics, aerobics machines, four times a week after work at a health club. She also plays tennis, backpacks, rafts, skis, and rock climbs!

Stress: Stress used to give Kay neck and back problems in her workaholic days. Exercise and a more reasonable work schedule have solved this problem.

Sleep: Seven hours "like a log."

Travel: About 25 percent of the year. When she travels, she tries to stay at hotels that have health clubs. "There's very little excuse for not getting your exercise when you're on the road," she says. Kay packs a leotard ("takes up no space") and a jump rope in case she's caught without proper facilities. She says you can do all you need to do right in your room.

Time Management: "There's time for everything you want to do if you manage your time! Otherwise it will get away from you." Her secrets? "I allot a certain amount of time to do each task, and I limit phone calls to a couple of minutes."

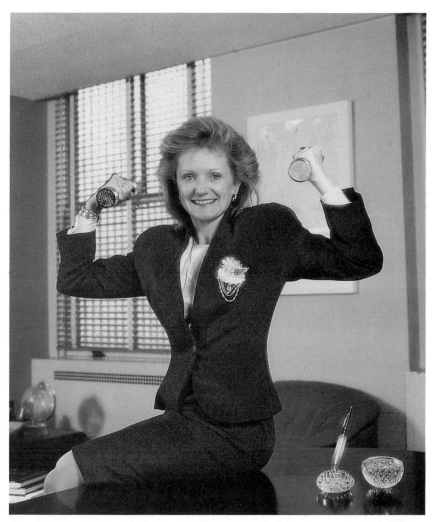

Kay Koplovitz, CEO and President of USA Network, finds that the mental stamina needed for white water river rafting and rock climbing translates to the boardroom.
(Photo by Kiki Bridges)

Positive Thinking: "A positive attitude goes a long way. I've always been positive."

Hobbies: White-water river rafting, rock climbing, tennis, cultural events.

To look at Kay's exercise repertoire, you would not be surprised to hear that her Walter Mitty dream is to be a world-class athlete (perhaps mountain climbing?). Kay is a superb athlete but jokes about being a bad swimmer. She says she would like to compete in a triathlon—"without the swimming part. I can't swim. I'd still be swimming when everyone else finished the event!" Kay does much better on the tennis court and, in fact, has competed in several tournaments.

In exercise, as in diet, Kay believes you must do what is best for you; there is no one formula that suits everyone. She says that if you are attuned to your body, "it will tell you what it wants."

On her way up the ladder, Kay pushed herself, often working from 8 A.M. to 1 A.M. One day, she realized that there was a diminishing return for her time after five o'clock. She remembers thinking, "This is crazy," and made a conscious effort from then on to make time for herself. Kay is convinced that long overtime hours of "pushing it" are unproductive and that it is better to go home and rest up for the next day.

Kay says her HealthStyle has "evolved over the past fifteen years" and that she now naturally prefers whole, fresh foods over the junk. She says that if you really want to lose weight, there are occasional sacrifices. You must say "There are things I like to eat but I'm just not going to eat them." Kay should know—she has had to work for her fitness and consequent health. Kay was an obese child who practically lived on ice cream and potato chips. And in college she went through the typical "eat as much pizza and drink as much beer as you can" phase. But finally, Kay got fed up (so to speak) and "went to my own school of discipline." She lost the weight and never went back. Her method is still the same—to simply cut back on foods rather than to go on some fanatical diet. "I'm not good at going home and weighing three ounces of this and that."

Kay started out to be a surgeon but has no regrets. She sees everything as experience. She thinks life is full of wonderful opportunities and chances and that we should expose ourselves to all we can. She fears upcoming students often measure success by dollars alone, which can create a one-dimensional point of view. Kay doesn't value as highly the individual who has tunnel vision. She thinks a broader scope benefits both your business and personal happiness. Kay believes it's important to think about social as well as business responsibilities. "Part of the reward of being successful is to be able to give something back."

EILEEN FORD
Chairman
Ford Models

Weight: Normal (but, "It depends on which day you're asking. But I have no use for the anorexic look—we call them 'X-rays'.")

Energy: "I'm very energetic naturally. I'm happy being busy. I'd probably be a meddlesome old lady if I weren't busy."

Diet: No sweet tooth, quit smoking thirty years ago, no caffeine, gives up alcohol when dieting. "If I have one glass of champagne, it goes right on the hips." Eats fish every day and rarely has meat. Grows her own vegetables.

Meals:
Breakfast—shredded wheat and fruit, an egg on weekends.
Lunch—fish and vegetables, also Chinese or Japanese food.
Dinner varies—sometimes a vegetable main dish, such as spinach/ricotta cheese mold, or salad with homemade dressing.

Favorite Foods: fish, Risotto al Fratia Dimare, crayfish cooked in dill, crystallized lemon and lime slices, any kind of chip. "I splurge in Paris and Rome—it's worth it."

Vitamins: C only.

Exercise: No regular program but occasionally uses an exercise bicycle in the morning when not traveling. Has other equipment, too, but admits: "You virtually never see me on any of them." Does back leg lifts and isometrics while conducting business around the office.

Stress: "I thrive on stress, I love chaos! I don't have time to worry about stress management."

Sleep: Four to five hours.

Travel: Seventeen weeks a year.

Time Management: "I lead a disorganized life. I have to be flexible from minute to minute. But I use my time very, very wisely. I budget it. I've even learned to dye my own hair! I'm very pleased with this latest accomplishment."

Positive Thinking: "I believe God put us on this earth with free will and the power to solve problems."

Hobbies: Gardening, theater, pets.

Eileen doesn't consciously work at a health program—she just does a lot of things right quite naturally. But she is human in regard to diet and has found that complete strangers feel it's their duty to keep the head of America's top modeling agency in line. "I was treating myself to a rare splurge—a bacon cheeseburger—when two women came up to me and said 'How *could* you!' " Eileen laughs as she also admits her secret desire is to "eat ten million pounds of potato chips."

Eileen's Walter Mitty dream is to be a big-band singer or to be in musicals. Realistically, Eileen says, she would have been a lawyer had things not turned out the way they did. She works with her husband and three of her four children and says she is content. In fact, she says, "I'll never retire—not until the kids kick me out!" Eileen loves animals and has two dogs, two cats and is "going to get a pig and a goat when I get my farm someday."

Eileen is a total pragmatist. She advises up-and-comers to "be very single-minded when you want to achieve something. You can't look right, you can't look left, and you can't look behind you. Just keep looking at what you're doing."

KATHRYN KLINGER
President
Georgette Klinger Cosmetics

Weight: 105–110 (5'4")

Married?: Yes, with two children.

Fitness Motivation: "I feel better when I'm exercising. It's an accomplishment when you feel yourself getting stronger." Also, "My husband is very active, and he shamed me into it." And if all else fails: "If you want to stay in shape, look at young girls and you should be inspired all the time. It's more of a battle the older you get."

Diet: "I talk about dieting more than I do it. Sugar is a weakness." Tips: "When you go to a restaurant, think ahead of time about what you're going to eat. Also, weigh yourself every day."

Meals:
Breakfast at 7:45 A.M.—juice and a high-fiber cereal.
Lunch—"Catch as catch can."
Dinner at 8—salad with everything on it and homemade dressing. "I'm either very good or very bad." She believes that "a big dinner will kill you."

Snacks: Snacks when she hasn't had a proper lunch.

Favorite Foods: Grapefruit, vegetables, chocolate.

Vitamins: No.

Exercise: "Exercise is my slice of time for me." Exercises three times a week before work—conditioning and toning with weights. Also takes tennis and karate lessons.

Stress: Rates her life as high stress but says that some stress is actually stimulating. She adds: "If I didn't do as much exercise as I do now, I wouldn't be able to cope with everything that goes on. It makes a big difference."

Sleep: Needs eight hours (says she looks better), usually gets six to seven.

Travel: At least six weeks a year. "I often use travel as a time to diet." She orders only nutritious, lo-cal meals and doesn't eat between meals.

Positive Thinking: "I work on positive thinking by talking to myself. You have to catch yourself thinking negatively and then talk to yourself."

Hobbies: Tennis, spending time with friends and child.

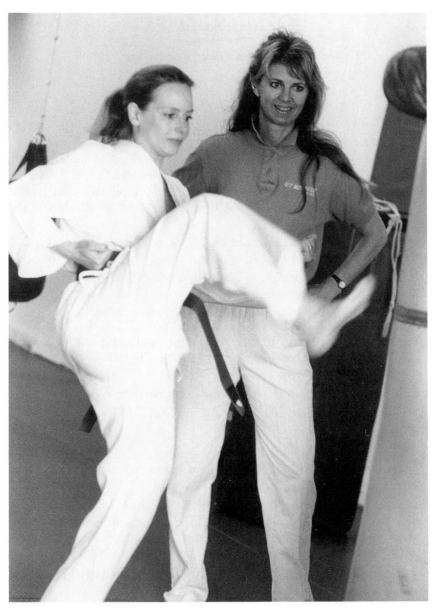

KRS watches as Kathryn Klinger, President, Georgette Klinger Cosmetics strengthens body and mind for her challenging day ahead. "Exercise is my slice of time for me."

A young working mother, Kathryn is doing it all, but fights time all the way. "From the minute I open my eyes in the morning it's—*Rush!*" In fact, she tries not to wear heels anymore, just so she can get around faster.

But Kathryn loves her life, and her advice is to "pick something you think you're going to like, because you're going to spend an awful lot of time doing it." She says if you don't like something, change it or ignore it but don't complain. She believes the same goes for exercise and diet: "If you don't like it, you won't stick with it."

Kathryn's Walter Mitty dream is to be a talk-show host, but she kids about her abilities in that area, saying, "God knows, we wouldn't have been able to afford anything!"

PAULA KENT MEEHAN
CEO, Chairman
Redken Laboratories

Age: 50s

Weight: 120

Married?: Yes. Husband is chairman of the board of Redken.

Energy: Genetically high. "But not as high as my mother's. She is eighty-six and goes to two parties a day."

Health-Oriented: "I'm mentally health-oriented."

Diet: "Low quantity, high frequency." (Doesn't skip meals.)

Meals:
   Breakfast—bran muffin, grapefruit.
   Lunch—tuna (health-oriented cafeteria at Redken).
   Dinner—chicken, dessert (see her special "Two-Minute Pie" in Chapter 11).

Favorite Foods: Chicken, chocolate brownies.

Vitamins: C, B12 (spray type).

Exercise: Walks three to four times a week (two miles). Stretches occasionally.

Stress: "I work very well under pressure. My mind seems to slow down if I don't have pressure."

Sleep: Nine hours. "I have to have my sleep."

Travel: Twenty trips a year (weekends mostly).

Positive Thinking: Yes. Her faith and meditation help, she says.

Hobbies: Work, reading.

"An all-American dream that is making a world of difference." Sounds like a commercial, but this is how a friend describes Paula. She says Paula is the true rags-to-riches story that can happen only in America. Raised in a poor family, Paula struck out to be a singer and actress and had some luck. She was the hat-check girl in the TV show *77 Sunset Strip* and also sang opera for seven years. When Paula did a Hamm's beer commercial that paid $3,000, she used the money to start building her dream—Redken. She had sensitive hair and skin (she was "broken off and broken out") and wanted a solution for herself and others with the same problems. Mounted at Redken is the oar she first used to mix ingredients in a bathtub.

Like Mary Kay (cosmetics) and Debbi Fields (cookies), Paula imparts an intimate family feel to her business. When the flu was going around, Paula personally distributed vitamin C to each employee with a note that said, "This is magic, and after you use it, you won't have any more colds or flu." It worked. One employee said that besides being a good boss, Paula is also a great spiritual example.

Paula is a risk-taker. She founded Redken in 1960, and in 1972 she was persuaded to go public. But she wasn't happy with the lack of control. "I wanted to come out with products at the right time for the right reasons, instead of trying to make quarterlies look good for the financial community." So, in November 1988 she put her neck (and pocketbook) on the line and bought back the company.

Although Paula thrives on pressure, she makes sure to get regular Saturday acupressure-type massages. She sometimes gets two a week if things are particularly high-paced.

Regarding diet, Paula advises people to "Forget the fanatical three-day-type diets. I've tried every one of them, and it's not the way to lose weight. The way to lose weight is over a three- to four-month period and changing your eating habits—and then *staying with* the change of habits."

MALCOLM STAMPER
President Emeritus
The Boeing Company

Weight: 195
Height: 5'11"

Meals:
   Breakfast—"We have a rack of whole-grain cereals; the latest is amaranth cereals" (a grain) with fruit juice instead of milk and sugar.
   Lunch—clear soup, tuna sandwich (dry), fruit.
   Dinner—fish (or chicken), vegetable, soup or salad (no dressing).
Favorite Foods: Home-grown vegetables, "Icebox Soups" (see following), peanut butter. Also, "I'm a sparkling water nut."
Favorite Recipe: Rye-oat bread. "You'd have to watch me to learn the recipe."
Vitamins: Multi, C.
Exercise: Jogs one hour, seven days a week. Also swims, skis, bikes and, oh yes, has climbed Mount Everest.
Stress: Exercise keeps him in balance.
Sleep: Four to five hours. "It's genetic. My mother says she doesn't sleep at all anymore, but I don't believe her."
Travel: Twelve weeks. "I carry food and water with me (Pritikin garlic pretzels, fruit, Perrier). In fact, the center section of my carry-on is filled with goodies."
Positive Thinking: "I'm wired positively."
Hobbies: Abstract artist, raises orchids, writes poetry.

––––––––––––––

The Man Who Built the 747

   Malcolm Stamper is a competitor all the way through. He has been in eight marathons, competed in the triathlete event, has won ski medals, has climbed Mount Everest, and has also won awards for his prize orchids (he tries to keep ten to twenty blooming in the house at all times).
   Mal calls his wife "the light of my life and the one who keeps me going in the athletic arena." Stamper was a college jock (football)

but proceeded to gain weight, drink, and smoke after college. When he married, his wife reintroduced him to fitness, and he has never turned back. Mal says she never nags, she just says, "Why don't we trek to the base camp of Mount Everest," and other fun-sounding things, so getting his body in shape again was initially just a means to an end.

When Mal started running with his wife, it was run/walk/run/walk. One day, he realized he'd run more than three miles without stopping and, competitor that he is, decided to enter his first race.

Besides his wife, Mal says his high school football coach inspired him the most. "He sort of made a man out of me—built my character and so forth." Mal went back to see him when he was out of shape, and his coach said, "You're in lousy shape." Mal said it didn't have an immediate effect, but it was instrumental in his "athletic comeback."

When it comes to diet, the Stampers are also "A" students. Mal's wife, daughter, and mother visited the Pritikin Longevity Center thirteen years ago to learn how to cook nutritiously. A few years ago, they all took a refresher course (along with twenty-four Boeing executives and their wives) that created a rededication to diet and nutrition. One tip: Stir fry with (de-fatted) chicken stock instead of with oil.

Mal enjoys spending time in the kitchen. He is famous for his "icebox soups" and his rye-oat bread. The soups are made with leftovers from the refrigerator. He puts the leftover steamed veggies through the food processor and adds raw ones for the texture. He adds them to chicken stock with some herbs, and voila—soups! Like Eileen Ford, Mal grows his own vegetables.

The rye-oat bread is another story. When Mal and his wife first married (during law school), his bride suddenly got recurrent headaches. Mal now jokes that the doctors assumed it was Mal that gave her the headaches, since he was the only new thing in her life. He tried changing his after-shave lotion and everything else—to no avail. It finally turned out to be an allergy to wheat. Mal said, "I was so thrilled it wasn't me that I learned how to make her a wheatless bread," which he still makes forty-three years later! He says he even takes the ingredients with them when they travel so he can make it on the road. Talk about true love. Some husbands can't even take a piece of bread out of the package and stick it in the toaster!

Mal's view of success is this: "It's no great accomplishment to be a financial success if you leave everything else behind." For example, he says, if you neglect your family, it will cause everybody mental stress. The trick is to keep everything in balance.

The son of farmers, Malcolm rates status and money low as reasons for working (passion and challenge rate high). He admits with a chuckle, however, that, "Power is good for leverage—it helped me put in running tracks at Boeing!"

As for retirement, Mal says, "I feel like I'm still in the process (of living)—I haven't written myself off yet. I don't say 'Gee, all this has happened, so now let's look back and reminisce.' You shouldn't think your life is over. You just go on to a greater challenge. You're still in the mainstream—it's just a matter of what are you going to do now. I'm sort of pleased with myself (particularly his work in developing the 747) but not overly satisfied. There's still a lot to be done." In fact among other things, Mal now runs a nonprofit publishing company called Story Tellers Ink, which prints books with a message for children.

One thing is certain, Mal likes to give back to the world. He is involved in the United Way and is interested in developing the talents of the needy and the handicapped. In addition, Mal sells his paintings for charities.

Mal's advice for CEOs-to-be: (1) Be flexible. Creativity is the ability to change. (2) Make an honest commitment. Don't say *if*. ("Like in a marathon, if you say, 'I don't know if I can run this, but I'll try'—you probably won't do it. Your body won't let you do it. Instead say, 'I'm *going* to run it.' The same goes with business goals.") (3) Communication. Always keep in mind how you are being heard and interpreted. Whether you're selling an idea or yourself, think of what they are hearing and what they need to hear.

Mal is an artist, an athlete, an inventor, a poet, a cook, a horticulturist, a humanitarian, a successful businessman, father, and husband. His own words perhaps describe him best: "Don't be afraid of failure—*Ski à la muerte!*" (*Ski to the death!*)

P.S.—Lunch came while we were talking (vegetable soup, wheat roll, nonfat milk, banana). I asked if the kitchen decided his menu for him. He laughed and said: "They know better. I say 'surprise me,' but I only give them a certain amount of latitude."

RANDY BARRON
President
Southwestern Bell Telephone Co.

Weight: 197
Height: 6'4"

Energy: "If I feel tired, I get up and walk around the block." Randy is also an expert cat napper.

Diet: "I can't remember the last time I had a 'full meal.' I don't go the mashed potatoes and gravy route."
Breakfast—bran muffin, V-8, decaffeinated coffee.
Lunch—soup, salad, or fish.
Dinner—fish or chicken, vegetable, salad.

Snack: Fruit, popcorn (no butter), "Randy's Go Juice" (see recipes in Chapter 11).

Favorite Foods: Fish, sauerkraut.

Vitamins: Multi, B, C, E, calcium.

Exercise: Runs or does weight machines one hour, six days a week, golfs (no cart).
Winter—uses treadmill indoors.

Stress: Exercise helps him. Has also studied meditation.

Sleep: Six to eight hours.

Travel: Twenty weeks. Travel interferes somewhat with his routine, but he tries to stay at a hotel with a gym or pool. If not, he jogs. Diet tip: Ask for a fruit plate or plain salad at convention meals.

Positive Thinking: Yes! Reads books on it (such as those by Norman Vincent Peale).

Hobbies: Fish, hunt, golf, woodworking. "Not enough time for everything."

———————

"I'm a health nut," professes Barron—and anyone who knows him would certainly agree. His wife, Marge, attests to Randy's high motivation level: "He reminds me to stay with the program."

Randy used to run in an old pair of basketball shoes long before running became the craze, no matter where he was (New Yorkers used to look at him strangely). He said he wasn't thinking about health so much back then—exercise just gave him "a high."

Randy believes that people owe themselves a well-cared-for-body, but he also believes that those who don't take care of themselves are cheating their families as well. Randy admits to being human when he says, "Some days I don't feel like doing it, but the very same time you don't feel good is when you've had a stressful day, and that's the very time you should be sure to exercise."

BRIAN DYSON
President, CEO Emeritus
Coca-Cola Enterprises

Weight: 160
Height: 6'2½"

Meals:
  Breakfast—cereal, toast.
  Lunch—salad plate, soup, yogurt.
  Dinner—stew, spaghetti.
Snack: Cookies.
Favorite Foods: Fish, salad, pasta with veal.
Vitamins: Multi, C (when he has a cold), Beta Carotene.
Exercise: Running, squash, tennis, racquetball, weights (two times a week, twenty minutes), swimming, skiing.
Sleep: Needs eight hours, gets six and a half, weekends nine.
Travel: Twenty weeks. It interferes with his routine but he sticks with it—running works almost anywhere, he says.
Positive Thinking: Yes. He is an optimist by nature but admits he must check himself on worrying.
Hobbies: Reads, "eclectic interest in everything," even tries short story writing.

———————

A funny, relaxed guy, Brian is a true health advocate. He has always been health-oriented, but got more so at age 43. However, he still eats red meat ("I'm from Argentina, where they eat lots of it").

Brian says he must have "good genes," because, while his diet is not immaculate (due to travel), he has immaculate vital statistics, including a good cholesterol ratio of about 3.0.

Brian is self-made, having grown up on a ranch in Argentina and leaving at 23 to make it in the Americas. He loves his work and says, "It's a sorry individual who is not doing the things that turn him on, after a certain level of success. There are dues to pay early in one's career," he adds, "but at a certain point, for the most part, one should be enjoying his work."

In life and business, Brian feels it's important to achieve objectives you've set, and to help build up other people. His motto:

"Look behind a good leader and see who follows—that defines a man's success at leadership." And always joking, he adds, "Behind every successful man stands an amazed mother-in-law."

A perfect Type B, Brian says that he's been happy at each level in his life. He works on the development of right brain/creative thinking.

FREDERICK RENTSCHLER
CEO, President Emeritus
Beatrice Companies

(Fred embarked on a complete HealthStyle program six years before this book was written. This profile includes a few before (THEN) and after (NOW) comparisons.

Weight: NOW—195
   THEN (Age 44)—245
Height: 6'
Cholesterol: NOW—185.
   THEN—250.

Energy: "Energy and enthusiasm have been two gifts I have been blessed with and that I have always used. But my best hours are from 6 A.M. to noon. I'm not a barrel of laughs after 10 P.M.—you better just put me to bed."

Meals: "It's more what I'm *not* eating than what I *am* eating."
   Breakfast—NOW: cereal, grapefruit juice (eggs two times a month), decaffeinated coffee.
            THEN: skipped breakfast or indulged in eggs, bacon, toast, and "the whole nine yards."
   Lunch—NOW: Open-face tuna sandwich with light mayonnaise, or chicken salad or fish, if dining out.
   Dinner—If home, frozen dinners (under 300 calories) or just a glass of 2 percent milk if he's really serious about dropping weight. If out, seafood, veal or chicken.
            THEN: Used to eat red meat fifteen times a week!
            NOW: Eats meat two or three times a week and never adds sugar or salt to anything.

Smoking: No. "I chewed cigars in the Marine Corps for effect, but it was just part of the staging."

Alcohol: NOW: No hard alcohol in six years. Drinks light beer and wine.
         THEN: Heavy scotch drinker.

Favorite Food: Chicken salad.

Favorite "Recipe": "My favorite recipe is whatever I have that's under 300 calories and takes six minutes in the microwave."

Vitamins: Occasionally.

Exercise: Treadmill four days a week, three miles at four MPH (forty-five minutes), golf.

Stress: "When I'm on the treadmill, an awful lot of anxieties just kind of melt away."

Sleep: Eight hours.

Travel: Twenty-seven weeks. Exercise is more difficult when he travels.

Hobbies: Fly fishing, golf, camping, horseback riding, hiking in Rockies.

Fred has a real rags-to-riches story in regard to fitness. He was fit when he was in the Marine Corps, but when he entered the business world, Fred became "a desk potato." On his way up the corporate ladder, Fred put all his energy and enthusiasm into his sedentary job, which required lots of travel. "Once you rivet your attention to the corporate ladder and goals and achievement in that sense, all else kind of goes away, including a hell of a good woman and a marriage. There were other sacrifices, including my body, which I just ignored going through the brass ring." He became overweight by eating the wrong foods and not exercising. Fred says he became health-oriented in the nick of time. "I think youth and good genes carried me through."

The turning point came six years ago. Fred was on a hunting trip with his best friend and mentor, the head of a multibillion-dollar company. The friend died of a heart attack during the outing. Coincidentally, the friend had been telling Fred about what he was going to do when he retired the following June—just five months away! He wanted to learn to fly fish, to improve his golf game, and to spend time with his grandkids. Fred said that his buddy ignored all the rules; he smoked, drank, ate poorly and was under a great deal of business-related stress.

Fred is happy to see more balance today with the young people. Couples are starting to share roles, including child rearing (Fred missed the opportunity to have children). Most important, he says, they seem to be enjoying themselves—*now.*

Fred's Walter Mitty dream is to be a cowboy and raise cattle in the high country, but he says he has no regrets, because he would always have wanted to succeed in the business world first, "as *I* measure success." Take note that Fred set his *own* standards for success. He did not chase after someone else's dream. And he adds, "I'll never have to wonder now when I'm on top of that horse in the mountains if I could have made it in the business world."

PAUL OREFFICE
Chairman of the Board
Dow Chemical

Weight: 182
Height: 6'

Meals:
  Breakfast—cereal, orange juice, English muffin.
  Lunch—soup, sandwich, fruit.
  Dinner—baked chicken, salad, vegetable, fruit.

Favorite Foods: Chicken, "all kinds of fruit," roast veal.

Favorite "Recipe": Salad dressing—"I make a big production out of it. I mix the pepper with the oil until it's dissolved and then the salt with the vinegar. I get pretty scientific."

Vitamins: Vitamin B (three times a day), C (2500 mg.), E (400 IU), calcium.

Exercise: Has not missed his daily workout in eleven years! His workout: forty minutes of pushups, chin-ups, leg lifts, back exercises, and LifeCycle. In addition, he walks two and a half miles several times a week and plays tennis for two hours four times a week.

Stress: "I pound the yellow ball" (tennis).

Sleep: Six to seven hours "like a baby."

Travel: Twenty weeks. "My workout may get modified to twenty-five minutes at times, but you make do."

Hobbies: Sports, activities with his children, plays cards, has written some music.

———————

Against All Odds would be the movie title I'd pick to depict the life of Paul Oreffice. An Italian immigrant, Paul came to America at 17. His father, Paul's greatest inspiration, was a fighter for freedom. As a child in Italy, Paul saw his father beaten in his quest and sent to jail. Paul says he learned at that early age how to be internally tough.

Paul entered Purdue University with no knowledge of the English language and calls it "the biggest challenge of my life." Eight

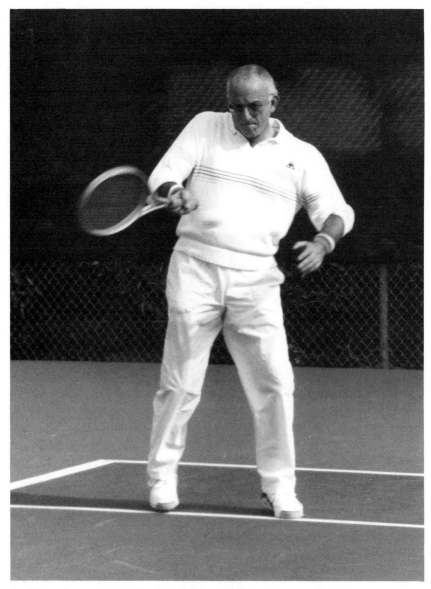

Applying a key success skill—focus—Paul Oreffice, Chairman of the Board, Dow Chemicals, says that to control stress, "I pound the yellow ball."

years later, at 25, Paul joined Dow Chemical as a sales trainee. By the age of 40, he held a top position at the firm. "My biggest talent has been in creating a good team and motivating others," he says.

Paul was always athletic as a youth (he played twelve sports in campus competitions!). Unfortunately, football gave him a serious knee injury. "After surgery, my doctor said I could never run again—and I believed him!" By the late 1960s, two things convinced Paul to change the course of his "no more running" fate. First, he decided he wanted to be active with his kids. Second, he took a long look in the mirror and saw a once-fit athlete now overweight and out of shape. "I couldn't have run to the corner," he confesses. So he had another surgery, followed it up with diligent exercise (100 leg lifts a day), and is now completely active. He lost thirty pounds and has kept it off. To maintain a good program, Paul says, "I believe consistency is important. Going on and off exercise with vacations, weekends, et cetera, does not work."

Regarding exercise, Paul and his wife are mutually supportive and enjoy walking and other activities together. Paul also loves to play tennis with his son. He jokes that he taught his son to play, and now Paul can't win a match against him. Had Paul not ended up as head of Dow Chemical, he believes he would have been a world-class bridge competitor. He has won the Spanish Open and Southwestern U.S. Championship titles and is a Life Master bridge player. Paul's only regret in life is not giving enough time to exercise in his twenties and thirties. Not surprisingly, his advice for upcoming CEOs (or anyone) is to *make* time for exercise. He knows it's possible, because he sees his son and others working extremely hard, but still finding time to stay fit.

BUILD MOMENTUM

Chapter Two

THE *HWW*
*H*EALTH*S*TYLE *T*EST
*H*OW *DO YOU MEASURE UP?*

Good health depends on genes or brains.
Don't bank on genes.
—*Raymond Hay, CEO emeritus, LTV*

Although America is in the midst of a consequential Wellness movement, opinions still vary widely about what exactly is "healthful" and what is not. Are those two eggs you had for breakfast really bad for you? Does snacking cause weight gain or can it help control weight and energy levels? How much good, if any, are your multivitamins doing you? These are just a few of the open issues in the health and fitness field today; issues that you should be able to discuss with your doctor.

Ask your doctor, but keep in mind that many physicians who are experts at diagnosis and treatment may be sadly behind the times when it comes to knowledge about nutrition, exercise and stress management. The nation's medical schools increasingly are being chastised for not placing more emphasis on the role of diet in disease prevention. Few doctors ask their patients about their eating habits during routine physical exams, yet more than half of their middle-aged patients have unhealthful cholesterol levels that are preventable through diet. The nation's medical profession also is sadly behind the times when it comes to knowledge about exercise and stress management. It shouldn't come as a surprise then to learn that the life expectancy for doctors is no higher than for other Americans.

So to whom can you turn? Whom should you believe? It's not an easy question, but in this book I give you a representative perspective by combining the most recent substantive findings with my original research. This information, along with the motivational skills and program guidance provided, will give you the foundation needed to become your own best expert and healer. The fact is, no one has the potential to be as tuned in to your inner processes as you yourself. The following test will give you a starting point as to your HealthStyle strengths and weaknesses. You can thus adapt the HWW HealthStyle Program to best suit your particular needs.

HOW DO YOU RATE?

How do you currently stack up against some of America's most successful people? You can quickly find out by taking the following HWW HealthStyle Test. The wellness rating I used is a synthesis of well-regarded data collected by those at the top of today's health fields, and some of the research on which it is based is examined more closely later on.

The people I interviewed were asked a total of seventy-two questions about their health practices. The test that you are about to take contains the key questions from those in-depth interviews. When you finish and compare your scores with those of the HWW leaders, you will have a clearer picture of where you excel and where you need to improve. This picture then will provide a baseline from which you can tailor your personal HWW HealthStyle Program.

Before you take the test, you should understand what your results will mean. Following is a slightly condensed version of the HWW Fitness Scale I developed. In this scale, the following ratings apply:

A = Very healthful
B = Fairly healthful
C = Inadequate or unhealthful

1. EXERCISE

A = more than two hours a week

B = one to two hours a week

C = less than one hour a week

Note: No particular type of aerobic exercise was considered superior to others, as long as a training heart rate (130 to 150 beats per minute) was achieved for periods of thirty minutes or longer.

2. FAT/OIL, SALT, SUGAR, AND RED MEAT

A = fewer than six servings total (all four categories) a day

B = six to twelve servings a day

C = more than twelve servings a day

A serving is considered to be one portion of a food that has a high content of any of the above. For instance, one helping of salty French fries or potato chips would be considered both a serving of salt and of oil. Adding salt to meat, or sugar or cream to coffee or cereal would also be considered as extra servings of salt, sugar, and fat, respectively.

3. CAFFEINE

A = fewer than two cups of coffee a day

B = two to five cups a day

C = more than five cups a day

4. ALCOHOL

A = fewer than two drinks a day

B = two to four drinks a day

C = more than four drinks a day

Note: A drink is defined as one beer, one glass of wine, or one ounce of hard liquor.

5. SMOKING

A = does not smoke

C = smokes

6. WEIGHT (see ideal weight table in the following chart)

A = within five pounds of ideal weight

B = within 10 percent over ideal weight

C = more than 10 percent over desirable weight

7. STRESS (see stress questions below)

A = score of −4 to 0

B = score of 1 to 4

C = score of 5 or more

The participants were asked the following three stress questions. Subtract the answer to Question 3 from the combined score of Questions 1 and 2.

(1) Rate the stress level of your job
(0 = no stress).   0 1 2 3 4

(2) Rate the stress level of your life other
than your job.   0 1 2 3 4

Men

Height	Small Frame	Medium Frame	Large Frame
5'1"	123–129	126–136	133–145
5'2"	125–131	128–138	135–148
5'3"	127–133	130–140	137–151
5'4"	129–135	132–143	139–155
5'5"	131–137	134–146	141–159
5'6"	133–140	137–149	144–163
5'7"	135–143	140–152	147–167
5'8"	137–146	143–155	150–171
5'9"	139–149	146–158	153–175
5'10"	141–152	149–161	156–179
5'11"	144–155	152–165	159–183
6'0"	147–159	155–169	163–187
6'1"	150–163	159–173	167–192
6'2"	153–167	162–177	171–197
6'3"	157–171	166–182	176–202

Women

Height	Small Frame	Medium Frame	Large Frame
4'9"	99–108	106–118	115–128
4'10"	100–110	108–120	117–131
4'11"	101–112	110–123	119–134
5'0"	103–115	112–126	122–137
5'1"	105–118	115–129	125–140
5'2"	108–121	118–132	128–144
5'3"	111–124	121–135	131–148
5'4"	114–127	124–138	134–152
5'5"	117–130	127–141	137–156
5'6"	120–133	130–144	140–160
5'7"	123–136	133–147	143–164
5'8"	126–139	136–150	146–167
5'9"	129–142	139–153	149–170
5'10"	132–145	142–156	152–173

Height without shoes, weight in pounds without clothes. From a table prepared by Metropolitan Life Insurance Company. Source of basic data: *Blind Study*, *1979*. Society of Actuaries and Association of Life Insurance Medical Directors of America.

(3) How well do you handle stress today
(0 = poorly)?   0   1   2   3   4

8. VITAL STATISTICS

Normal clinical ranges for both men and women are:

Cholesterol   120–275

HDL (high density lipoproteins)   29–77

Blood pressure   ideal ratio: 3 to 2   (120 over 80)

Note: "Normal clinical ranges" can vary somewhat from laboratory to laboratory. The term simply means the average scores of samples that have come through that particular lab; "normal" doesn't mean healthy. As you now know, the average "normal" population is not considered optimum by any means. Thus, the following breakdown:

Cholesterol:

A = 120 to 199

B = 200 to 239

C = over 239

HDL:

A = 70 or higher

B = 50 to 69

C = below 50

Blood pressure ratio (systolic over diastolic):

A = 3 to 2 within 5 points

B = 3 to 2 within 10 points

C = over 10 points difference from 3 to 2

Taking the HWW HealthStyle Test

To find out how you measure up now against America's top executives, take the HWW HealthStyle Test that follows. Later, when you have made some needed changes to your HealthStyle, take the test again and see how you are progressing.

The HWW HealthStyle Test

1. How many hours a week do you exercise?   _____

2. Do you exercise consistently—at least three times a week for thirty or more minutes per session?   Yes _____ No _____

3. Are you over your ideal weight?
   (See preceding chart)   Yes _____ No _____

4. By how many pounds?   _____

5. How many servings daily do you
   typically have of the following?
   (as per previously mentioned serving
   description)

Fat, oils	0	1	2	3	4+
Salt	0	1	2	3	4+
Sugar	0	1	2	3	4+
Red meat	0	1	2+		
Caffeine	0	1	2	3	4+
Alcohol	0	1	2	3	4+

6. Do you eat breakfast?   Yes _____ No _____

7. Do you eat dinner before 7:30 P.M.?
   (or at least three hours before retiring)   Yes _____ No _____

8. Do you smoke?   Yes _____ No _____

9. Do you regularly apply a specific
   technique to handle stress (meditation,
   positive thinking, etc.)?   Yes _____ No _____

10. Rate the stress level of your job
    (0 = none, 4 = high):   0 1 2 3 4

11. Rate the stress level of your life other
    than your job: 0 1 2 3 4

12. How do you handle stress today?
    (0 = poorly)   0 1 2 3 4

13. Rate the extent to which you enjoy your
    job: (0 = no enjoyment)   0 1 2 3 4

14. Would you do your job for free?
    (financial considerations aside)   Yes _____ No _____

15. Vital statistics:

    Blood pressure   _____
    Cholesterol   _____
    HDL (High Density Lipoproteins)   _____

Scoring Yourself

QUESTION NUMBER:

1. Over two hours = 15 points, one to two hours = 10 points, under
   one hour = 0 points.

2. Yes = 10 points.

3. No = 15 points (see ideal weight ranges, page 36).

4. Subtract two points per five pounds. (One point per 2 1/2 pounds)

5. Subtract 1 point per serving, but subtract 8 points total for a 4+ daily intake of fat, salt, sugar and caffeine, and subtract 8 points total for 2+ servings of red meat. Subtract 15 points total for 4+ servings of alcohol.

6. Yes = 5 points

7. Yes = 5 points

8. Subtract 20 points if you smoke.

9. Yes = 5 points.

10. Subtract the number of points circled.

11. Subtract the number of points circled.

12. Add twice the number of points circled.

13. Add the number of points circled.

14. Yes = 8 points.

15. Vital statistics: Add 1 point if you know any or all of your scores. Add 8 points for each vital statistic within normal range (refer to vital statistic ranges). Add no points if you don't know what your statistics are.

Rating Your Score

87–100	Excellent!
73–86	Good
60–72	Fair
40–59	Poor
0–39	Very Poor

Compare Your Scores with the Leaders

AVERAGE TOTAL SCORE:

The HWW Males	The HWW Females
90	81

The HWW "A" HealthStyle Profile

What did it take, in my study, to be rated "healthy"? When the test scores were all in, those who received "A" marks had the qualities listed below. These men and women also had a "healthy attitude," meaning they were consciously committed to better health and practiced regular health habits. One way you can get started toward a better HealthStyle is to draw from the experiences and examples of the successful people in this book and adapt some of their practices to your own lifestyle. They pursue a lifestyle that combines regular physical activity with sensible eating, and they achieve healthy, successful results.

THE HWW "A" HEALTHSTYLE PROFILE

1. Exercises regularly two hours or more a week.
2. Weight is within ideal range.
3. Eats little fats, oils, sugar, salt, and red meat.
4. Drinks fewer than two cups of coffee a day.
5. Drinks fewer than two alcoholic beverages a day.
6. Does not smoke.
7. Has a low level of stress.
8. Has a cholesterol range of 120 to 199.
9. Has an HDL level of 70 or higher.
10. Has a blood pressure ratio of 3 to 2 within 5 points.

NO
GUILT

Chapter Three

FOOD STRATEGIES

THE BOTTOM LINE ON EATING RIGHT

Fitness and good eating are addictions, and I'm hooked. The healthier you are, the higher you are. A lot of people never know what that feels like.

— Gilda Marx, CEO, Gilda Marx Industries

Eating right is not always easy in this "fast-forward" world. Still, the leaders I interviewed have developed successful strategies for eating the right foods in appropriate quantities, even during the course of a very challenging day. You can easily adapt some of their winning strategies to your own HWW HealthStyle Program and start eating healthier today.

WHY EATING LIKE "EVERYBODY ELSE" CAN MAKE YOU GAIN WEIGHT

Most Americans are overweight. In fact, more than seven out of ten Americans are over their recommended weight. One in five is considered obese (weighs 20 percent more than his or her ideal weight). And things are getting worse, not better. The average American gains weight annually. We weigh an average of six pounds more today than we did in the 1960s, and we eat 10 percent more than we did in the 1970s. This news becomes particularly mind boggling when you realize that, at any given time, approximately 50 percent of American women and 25 percent of men are on a weight-loss diet.

How do we gain this weight? We consume more per capita than any other country, including a typical daily intake of twenty-four teaspoons of sugar, three cups of coffee, and two to three ounces of alcohol (we also smoke one pack of cigarettes a day). Did I include fats? We each eat an average of six pounds of potato chips a year. Apparently the "health craze" sweeping the country is not exactly fanatical.

Americans are notorious breakfast and lunch skippers. With all these missing meals, you'd think we'd at least compare favorably to the HWW leaders in terms of weight, but this is not the case. *The average American male weighs nearly twelve pounds more than the HWW male of his same height.* Specifically, we eat nearly twice as many desserts as they do. On the other hand, they eat nearly twice as much of the fiber food—cereal—as the rest of us. They also eat far more of the "brain/heart food"—fish—than the rest of us.

I often beg my clients to treat themselves at least as well as they treat their pets. I was talking with a friend I hadn't spoken with for awhile and asked about her cat. "Old Sprouty?" she asked in a resigned tone. "Oh, we just feed him diet cat food and hope for the best." When I finished laughing, it occurred to me that Sprouty was probably being treated better than most people treat themselves. Diet cat food would probably be an improvement for most of us.

The following chart will give you some eye-opening comparisons between the food consumption of the general population and that of the men and women I studied.

**Daily Food Consumption of the HWW Leaders
Compared with the General Population**

Food	General Population, %	HWW Leaders, %
(one or more servings)		
Meat/Poultry	86	46
Fish/Shellfish	1.2	64
Eggs	16.2	7
Fruits/Vegetables	55	97
Cereals	18.8	57
Dessert	43.1	5.5

The general population eats more meat, less fish, more eggs, less cereal (fiber), many more desserts and, sadly, much less fruit and vegetables than the HWW leaders. MRCA Information Services has found that Americans eat an average of 236 eggs a year. The number of eggs, however, bothers me less than the way we eat them—most of us (65 percent) prefer them scrambled or fried. According to the National Cancer Institute, on a given day, 45 percent of the people who took part in the National Health and Examination Survey ate *no* fruit or fruit juice, and 48 percent ate *no* vegetables (or only one serving, which included fried potatoes).

While most people seem to start putting on weight at around age 30 to 40, the men and women in my study saw that weight gain as a personal red flag and took measures to stop it.

Bob Wycoff, president of Atlantic Richfield, says he became health conscious in his thirties and became more serious about it in his forties. Still maintaining that program in his sixties, Wycoff exercises at least four times a week, doing calisthenics and the stair machine at the local YMCA. And at the top of his favorite food list are grapefruit and chicken! Most Americans, on the other hand, don't perceive a little weight gain as particularly significant and allow the situation to continue—or don't have the proper knowledge or motivational tools to make weight loss *stay* lost. In fact, it is said that 75 to 95 percent of us will regain the weight we worked so hard to lose. And, according to The Washington *Post*, only 1 in 200 will keep the weight off for more than five years.

By incorporating the mindset that is part of the HWW Program, however, you can learn to automatically spot these red flags as they come up and know what to do about them.

EATING HABITS OF AMERICA'S MOST SUCCESSFUL

"Diet is the hardest—I've been plump all my life," says Mary Kay, founder and chairman of Mary Kay Cosmetics. Mary Kay stays in control of what she calls her "plump genes" (so they don't become "fat genes") by weighing herself on a scale first thing each morning. If she's one pound over her limit, "the next day is dieting." This strategy works for her; she has worn the same dress size for twenty-five years.

"I think about 'no no' foods too much," admits Richard Mahoney, CEO of Monsanto. Mahoney says he now eats right most of the time, but still occasionally splurges on pizza with his kids on weekends. For him, getting some expert help on changing his diet worked: his weight is down and holding.

The HWW leaders readily admit to eating the foods of mortals, including burritos, fried chicken, chocolate chocolate-chip ice cream, pastries in Paris . . . you name it. But they allow these temptations to creep into their diets only on occasion—as a brief change of pace.

Having more than an occasional treat of these foods, the HWW leaders have seen, quickly leads to weight gain.

Weight gain also can rear its head when major life changes occur. For example, Columbe Nicholas developed weight problems after she left a physically active retailing career for her post as president of Christian Dior, where she spent more time working at a desk. First thing she knew, she'd gained 10 pounds. "I went to a nutritionist who did some modification to change my eating habits," she says, "like not being a member of the clean-plate club." She adds that she learned "it takes changing a pattern of eating habits to make a consistent change in one's weight." Now, she says, her improved eating habits come naturally.

Lucky Stores CEO and chairman Larry DelSanto never had a weight problem until he moved to San Francisco and dined out on pizzas and hot dogs while his wife, who helps maintain dietary order for him, wrapped up the sale of their home in Illinois. To his surprise, he gained 25 pounds, and his cholesterol rose 30 points. His wife finally joined him and helped him get his diet back on track. He soon lost the weight and lowered his cholesterol back to normal. He now avoids dietary temptation at the office by keeping plenty of fresh produce around, rather than pastries and other traditional workplace snack foods.

Continental Groups CEO emeritus, Bruce Smart, Jr., is another believer in home cooking and makes an effort to eat at home whenever possible. In fact, this is one area where most of the males have an advantage over the females. Most wives of the men in my study are also health-oriented, so the men have the added bonus of homemade, healthful meals on a regular basis. Bruce says, "My wife is an excellent cook—interesting meals without being unhealthful."

To get their HealthStyles to where they are today, most of the HWW men and women have had to reeducate themselves and break deeply ingrained habits. They have no miracle "skinny genes"; when they behave like the general population they reap the same results: weight gain and stress. As children, the majority were taught to drink their (high-fat) milk and eat everything on their plates, which usually included plenty of red meat, potatoes, and gravy. And when their plates were clean, they were rewarded with cake and ice cream. If they were a little thick around the middle, it was simply regarded as a sign of vitality. Robert McCowan of Ashland Oil grew up during the Depression, when "fat meant prosperity." Like many of his peers, he was encouraged to clean his plate. He says he had to change many of his eating habits as an adult. When we first spoke a few years ago, McCowan told me about his roller-coaster struggle with weight. He said he had closets full of clothes in five sizes, from A to E. Since then he has stabilized into the A-size closet, firmed up his stomach muscles and keeps his cholesterol under 200. McCowan says, "If you don't have control over your body, you have no control over other things."

While you may not be a member of the Clean Plate Generation, if you are a member of the generations that followed you know that eating habits are not much better. Among other things, we are growing up on TV, subjected to 20,000 ads for food each year.

Unfortunately, the conveniences of modern technology have also become our foes. Household appliances and advanced transportation have gradually and quite insidiously made us less and less active and have thus taken a toll on our health. With the advent of dishwashers, washing machines, electric mixers, vacuum cleaners, and other "helpers," a woman who consumes 2,400 calories today (as she typically did in the Thirties) will gain weight rapidly, unless she is in training for a decathlon. To maintain weight today, most white-collar men must limit their daily intake to 2,000 to 2,400 calories, and most women can eat only 1,800 calories a day (that's a hamburger with the works, potato chips, and a piece of chocolate cake).

Do these "captains of industry" crave sweets? The women do, the men don't. Debbi Fields likes to snack on candy and taste-test her own cookies. Atlantic Richfield's Camron Cooper says she also loves Mrs. Fields' cookies. Gilda Marx is also a cookie lover, while Mary Kay (of Mary Kay Cosmetics) prefers candy and cake. Marcia Israel (of Judy's clothing stores) is tempted by desserts and candy, but it is an urge she curtails pretty well (except for the candy in Hong Kong, because "it's so good"). Redken's CEO and founder, Paula Kent Meehan, keeps her weight in check by eating a good roughage breakfast (grapefruit and a bran muffin) and no snacks, but she allows herself dessert with dinner: "Dessert is my reward!" she says.

How do they have their cake and eat it, too, without becoming MooMoo Mamas? In a word—moderation. This is an easy word to throw around, but a hard one to apply. The women in my study want their sweets, but also want to keep their figures, so they have developed their own strategic balance of reward and discipline. Debbi Fields says that she must occasionally eat sweets, or she will binge on them sooner or later. "I've learned to eat the foods I love and leave the rest. I've tried every diet under the sun, but I have to follow what I enjoy." Debbi Fields' own customized diet formula is as follows:

1. Include some sweets.
2. Weigh daily.
3. Eat less in general.
4. Refuse to buy larger size clothes. ("That's my weight control secret.")

This formula works for Debbi, but may be ineffective for others. Armco's Bob Boni, for example, thinks playing with sweets can get sticky (in more ways than one). "It's easy to delude oneself into believing that a little dessert won't hurt or that a few days missed exercise is not a calamity. The challenge, of course, is to get back on course." I relate Debbi's story, however, to demonstrate how programs must be individualized. While I do not advocate sugar, I have worked with many people who won't or can't give it up and still have had success in losing weight. One client, a busy executive, recently lost 90 pounds. We worked her daily sweet "fixes" into her program (one or two small cookies, for example) which she said took away the trapped, ascetic feelings of "dieting," and her weight loss was relatively painless. For others (myself included), complete abstinence from sugar is necessary. To some of us, it is a harmful allergy food, even in small doses. With abstinence, the ongoing daily battle of "Should I? Shouldn't I" is eliminated. Instead, there is just *one* decision *one* day. And mercifully, abstinence gets easier the longer you abstain. The HWW Diet & Nutrition Program will help you with moderation, bingeing and other weight sabotagers.

How Your Personal Stats Can Motivate You

Chevron's James Sullivan says he has a built-in weight motivator: his blood pressure. When his weight goes up, his blood pressure goes up. James refuses to go on blood pressure medication as long as he knows he can control it. So, when he's up a few pounds, he says he immediately cuts back on food portions and drops the pounds, as well as his blood pressure.

Even though exercise is her career, Gilda Marx also must watch the scale. She admits, "I have to watch my weight, because I have a healthy appetite for healthy food. A lot of people don't understand that you can't eat *all* the salad you want; you can only eat so many calories a day. I think many people who are heavy just don't know when they are full."

"Just eating right won't make you CEO of a company," adds Columbe Nicholas of Christian Dior, "but it shows a discipline that carries over to the workplace." Philip Smith of General Foods has this kind of dietary discipline. At age 53, he runs 25 miles a week and puts in 2-½ hours a week in the gym, in addition to tennis, skiing, and wind surfing. Nonetheless, Philip still has to watch his weight. He keeps his weight down when he's on the road by eating only half of each meal, rather than using travel time as binge time. Philip knows he has to face the scale, so he compensates accordingly. Others mentioned similar tricks.

Kathryn Klinger of Georgette Klinger Cosmetics doesn't mince words: "If you're a woman who's past a certain age, you're on a diet." It's just one of those facts that must be faced. For most people, that "certain age" is between thirty and forty. And sure enough, that's the age when the majority of the individuals I studied had to get serious about watching their weight. Personal stats keep them motivated.

WHAT YOU DON'T KNOW CAN HURT YOU

Today's medical professionals are woefully undereducated in preventive medicine, but they are undeniably invaluable to us and shouldn't shoulder all the blame for our ignorance. Advertisers for food products don't exactly make eating right a "piece of cake" and should assume a more informed and informative role. For instance, "no cholesterol" on labels doesn't mean that there aren't any artery-clogging saturated fats. Most "no cholesterol" dairy substitutes are very high in saturated fats. Also, "low fat/2 percent" milk is 2 percent fat by weight, but it really has 35 percent saturated fat by calories, which is not much better than whole milk with 48 percent of its calories from fat (anything over 30 percent is considered a high-fat food). *Non*fat milk is 2 percent saturated fat by calories and is a better choice to pour over your unsugared, high-fiber cereal (or, better yet try the Yogurt Milk in Chapter 11). Unfortunately, there are more Americans who drink whole milk than those who drink low-fat and nonfat combined.

Along with misleading advertising, we also must deal with the seemingly ever-changing facts. Yes, it can be discouraging trying to keep up with the latest nutritional advice, especially when it abruptly changes after you've been denying yourself certain foods for the past year. "What? Now you say I *can* eat eggs?" You feel so cheated, so deceived.

Oat bran is a good example of a nutritional buzz word that went to the hype limits. When I started seeing oat bran in junk food (chips), I knew overkill had hit. And why was oat bran so hot? Because of an even bigger buzz word, the biggest of the past decade: cholesterol. The history of cholesterol do's and don'ts epitomizes the "now this, now that" syndrome. Trying to figure out what to do can be confusing. And I say this based on my discussions with one of the world's leading experts on cholesterol and heart disease, Dr. William Castelli, medical director of the Framingham Heart Study. According to Dr. Castelli, contradictory interpretations of clinical trials and population studies have made it difficult for the general population to get clear answers regarding (among other things) the cholesterol problem. So it's no wonder we're confused.

So what do you do? How do you handle the changes in what is—or is not—good for you? What you *don't* do is say, "Who knows what to eat—one day it's this and another day it's that. So, I just eat the same old things, and I'm still alive." Needless to say, this is not a constructive response. Instead, listen to the latest findings, do a little investigating, and follow your gut instinct about what is good or bad for you. Finally, take the newest advice or recommendations in small doses and see how it feels. If and when a certain claim to which you have been fervently adhering is disproved, bypass feeling foolish, helpless, or angry, and shift course along with science. *Be flexible.*

One thing is clear from my study and other studies, however. Overall refinement of your dietary intake *does* make a difference. By maintaining proper weight, reducing the amount of animal fats you eat, and eating whole grains, you can reduce your chances of getting cancer by 50 percent. Eating more fruits and vegetables will also reduce cancer risks, since they contain antioxidants that guard against cancer-causing free radicals. Eliminating fatty animal products from your diet can cut your risk of heart disease by 88 percent and also significantly reduce your chances of getting rheumatoid arthritis. Among other things, fish can reduce the blood fat triglyceride. Eating just one serving of fish a week reportedly lowers a man's risk of heart disease by 36 percent and two servings can lower it by 64 percent. Simply losing weight will lower your blood pressure. Soluble fibers (specifically gums, pectin, and lignin) prevent or reduce the absorption of certain substances (such as cholesterol and glucose) into the bloodstream. The benefits are lower cholesterol levels and steadier blood sugar levels, which offset hypoglycemic tiredness and low energy. Soluble fiber foods include grapefruit, oat bran, cabbage, broccoli, apples, carrots, and beans.

Not surprisingly, the HWW leaders don't follow a rigid "meal plan" per se, and you needn't either. While you need to be aware of what goes into your body by checking food labels for such substances as hidden sugar, fat, or preservatives, this process can be taken too far. Analyzing and accounting for every gram of fat, fiber, protein, carbohydrate, and sodium ingested can become an obsession to some and discourage others. Frankly, the people I studied don't have the time to do this, and I'm sure you don't either. Their strategy has been to *simplify* and shorten the time and energy they spend achieving their dietary goals. It should not only be easy to eat right, but it should also be enjoyable. The men and women in this book are not into deprivation. They enjoy the foods they eat, and I have confidence that you will enjoy eating healthier, too. In other words, you should be aware of basic dietary guidelines, but you don't have to become a scientist to eat correctly.

There is no such thing as *the* perfect weight-loss diet or nutritional "itemized" diet that can be applied to everyone. There are just too many individual factors that must be taken into account, such as physiological (digestion) and psychological differences. For example, because each digestive tract has different absorption abilities and varying availability of enzymes, "Two people eating the same diet may end up with dramatically different intakes of protein, carbohydrate or other nutrients," according to author Rudolph Ballentine, M.D., in *Diet & Nutrition*. Ballentine also believes that, unfortunately, neither the science of nutrition nor the general public is geared toward mental-nutritional interplay. The computer-analyzed and prescribed diet program craze aptly demonstrates this point. Ballentine says this approach "totally ignores the importance of the mind and the effect of one's mental and emotional habits on nutritional requirements." Computer programs overlook personal awareness, "body feel," and the ability of one's psychological state to affect the way he or she absorbs and metabolizes food.

So, which weight loss program *should* you follow? *Not* one that prescribes identical food lists for everybody. Once you have experienced the Diet & Nutrition Program and the Speed Cooking Plan in Chapter 11 for 60 to 90 days, you will understand the concept of dietary and nutritional evolution and will be able to continue the process for a lifetime.

ALL YOU NEED TO KNOW ABOUT WATER: DRINK IT!

Soft drinks now have overtaken water as the number-one thirst quencher in the United States. As treats, soft drinks are fine, but they are not a replacement for the recommended six to eight cups of water a day (nor is coffee, juice, or herbal tea, for that matter). Keep a bottle of water in your car and another one on your desk. Then get in the habit of *drinking* those bottles every day. Squeeze a lemon into the water for a great-tasting, detoxifying drink. Go one step further and add powdered vitamin C to your water and get "vitamized" all day long (use a colored bottle to protect the C from being broken down by sunlight).

Water balances body chemistry, helps eliminate fat, maintains muscle tone, and prevents sagging skin that follows weight loss. Many report increased energy with their increased water intake. Kathryn Klinger says, "I often find when I'm sort of tired, I'm really actually thirsty." If you don't drink enough water, your body actually retains more water as a survival mechanism. So if you tend to retain water, drink more water and that bloated feeling will decrease, along with the extra pounds. Water can often relieve constipation within about an hour—drink four to six glasses of water and wait. Keep a bottle of water by your sink and drink it while getting ready for work, as part of your morning routine.

A final water tip: Drink water (or any liquid) no sooner than half an hour before a meal and at least a half hour to an hour after a meal. Try this for three weeks. You'll get used to it, and this schedule will give your digestive enzymes a chance to go to work undiluted by the water, which might alleviate the tiredness you may feel after meals. Remember, it's important to think of your new habit in positive terms—drinking water *adds* energy as opposed to being one more "must do" in life. Make a water commitment of one glass (8 ounces) a day for the first week, two glasses the second week, and so on until you are up to six to eight glasses a day. If that rate is too fast for you, set your own rate, but be specific about your resolution or it won't happen. You will notice more energy, a glowing complexion, and very grateful intestines.

GOOD NEWS ABOUT EGGS

Eggs have had bad press. For people who are not genetically prone to high cholesterol (10 to 15 percent of the population), there is no reason to be egg phobic. The National Cholesterol Education Program even admits that cutting down on dietary cholesterol "gets variable results." Further, egg lecithin is fast gaining recognition for its health benefits and is even being sold as a nutritional replacement therapy for the negative effects of envelope viruses (including Epstein Barr Syndrome and AIDS), although no formal claims can be made at this point. While eggs contain cholesterol, they actually contain minimal saturated fat, making them one of the few high-quality proteins low in fat and calories. Egg whites are one of the highest quality, undiluted proteins that you can eat. So if you are interested in local, no cholesterol protein, substitute two egg whites for one whole egg in recipes and make omelettes with the egg whites (the cholesterol and calories are in the yolk).

It was once suggested to avoid eggs altogether, then two eggs a week became acceptable, then three, and now four eggs a week are considered "safe." Until further "official notice," you should continue practicing egg discretion, but I must admit that it wouldn't surprise me one day to read: "NEWS FLASH—EGGS ARE GOOD FOR YOU!"

BAD NEWS ABOUT SUGAR

Here's another newsflash for you: "LOSE WEIGHT AND GAIN ENERGY—QUIT EATING SUGAR!" Sounds like one of those ads for another oddball diet, but this is one headline that would be worth heeding. Granted, it's not an easy task, since we're a nation addicted to sugar. We each eat 133 pounds of sugar a year (including all sources of sugar). That's about two and a half pounds of sugar a week! In fact, sugar constitutes 20 to 25 percent of all calories ingested, or about 500 to 600 calories a day. You're probably thinking, "Gee that's a lot. I wonder who's eating my share?" Surprise, it's probably you. Sugar is everywhere—in hamburger buns, ketchup, salad dressing (even diet brands), bread, and other foods.

In spite of the health movement, ice cream is making a comeback with the American public. Even though it is high in sugar, fat, and calories, consumption has more than doubled in the past few years. One woman's magazine even featured an ice cream diet! (Notice how a part of you wants to run out and try it—yet another painless "miracle cure.") If you crave something cold and sweet, try nonfat frozen yogurt, glacé, or gise. Give yourself a month or so to adjust, and it will taste just as good to you. (Remember this crucial timeline about addictions—the first twenty-one days of starting or stopping anything are the roughest, but it does get easier.)

Refined sugar has no vitamins, digestible minerals, enzymes, trace elements, fiber, or protein. But sugar does have calories. In other words, it's useless but not harmless. Sugar can trigger diabetes, arteriosclerosis, hypoglycemia, depression, and other illnesses. Sugar reduces the amount of energy available to muscles and can cause a chromium deficiency, which can lead to diabetes and heart disease. Ingesting sugar before exercise can reduce endurance up to 19 percent. It can also cause the release of endorphins, resulting in the well-known sugar "high" (and a desire for even more sugar). Get your endorphin high from exercise. It's safer. (More on endorphins later.)

Unfortunately, statistics say we are shifting from sugar to sugar substitutes. Studies report that people who use sugar substitutes tend to be overweight or to gain more weight than nonusers, perhaps because sugar substitutes may stimulate hunger. And should I even begin harping about the chemicals in these substitutes? No need—that's old news, right? For sweetening, try substituting Dr. Bronner's Barleymalt Sweetener (powdered), which is delicious (ask for it at health food stores). It is low calorie and actually good for you.

SEPARATING PROTEIN FROM FAT

Americans rank first in the world in meat consumption. In 1989, we each ate an average of a half pound a day or 218.4 pounds for the year. That translates to 56 ounces a week, compared to nine ounces per week consumed by the men and women in this book. You really shouldn't eat red meat more than about once a week, because it contains too much saturated fat. Lean meat isn't the perfect solution, either; it contains as much cholesterol as fatty meats (cholesterol is found in the lean tissue, not the fat). Also, you should avoid most processed meats such as hot dogs or packaged luncheon meats because they contain known carcinogens and most have a very high fat content of around 80 percent. Some advertise lower fat content, but watch for sodium and preservatives. Unfortunately, Americans eat even more processed meat than they do regular red meat.

Will you be missing anything if you don't eat any red meat? Red meat does contain the hard-to-find vitamin B12, but you can get your quota from fish and dairy products.

Too much protein of any kind can cause calcium depletion (even with calcium supplementation), because so much calcium is needed to offset the acidifying effect of sulfur-containing amino acids. Translation: too much protein can contribute to osteoporosis. How much protein should we consume? About 15 percent of our total caloric intake. If you have a desire to know the exact amount, multiply your weight times 0.36 (Example: 150 lbs. × 0.36 = 54 grams of protein per day).

We should lower our cheese consumption, as well. Most Americans eat more than 25 pounds of cheese a year—more than double the intake of the 1960s. Hard cheese contains more saturated fat than beef and is very high in calories. One ounce (a 1-inch cube) of cheddar cheese has about two and a half teaspoons of fat! Fortunately, there are now some improved low-fat, low-sodium cheeses available that are especially good for cooking or eating at room temperatures (Light Vitalait by Cabot Farmer's Co-op is a good one). A better, leaner source of protein is chicken with the fat and skin removed. But the best source of animal protein by far is delicious, inexpensive fish. There's such a variety of fresh fish available in this country; it's one of our great natural resources (see Chapter 11 for easy cooking tips). While fish does not directly lower total cholesterol levels, it can help prevent cholesterol and blood platelets from clogging your arteries.

To help you modify your own diet, the relative amounts of saturated fat and cholesterol of a few high-protein foods are listed below. Watch the saturated fat, perhaps a bigger culprit than cholesterol.

	Cholesterol, mg	Saturated Fat, g
Egg	213	2
Cheddar Cheese (3 oz.)	90	18
Lean Skinless Chicken (or Turkey, 3 oz.)	66	0.9
Halibut (3 oz.)	35	0 (trace)
Lean Beef (18% fat) (3 oz.)	73	8

By the way, vegetarians have lower blood pressure, are less prone to osteoporosis, have better total cholesterol and HDL scores, and decreased cancer risk. But don't think of vegetarianism as the ultimate goal—very few of the people I studied are vegetarians.

THE BOTTOM LINE ON FATS AND OILS

Remember that fat is the enemy of fitness: it slows digestion, thickens blood, and reduces the amount of oxygen reaching body tissues. Fats and sugars compromise IMMUNITY, accelerate aging, and displace vitamins and minerals from your diet. Beware of hidden fats (as well as sugars and calories) that spoil the best intentions of eating right. Mayonnaise is 100 calories a tablespoon—fat and sugar— that can add up to just about a pound of weight gain a month (at the rate of one tablespoon a day). The slimming effect of a salad can be spoiled by high-fat, sugary salad dressings. And as pointed out by Charles Kittrel of Phillips Petroleum, "Even fish can be deadly with all those sauces." So pay attention to detail in the food you eat.

Cholesterol is a dirty word to most Americans, but as I've pointed out, the real enemy now is saturated fat. Saturated fats come from animal products and plant oils that are solid at room temperature. According to the American Heart Association, our daily diet should not contain more than 22 grams of saturated fat, or 67 grams total fat intake. Experts say you can actually become obese on as little as 1,500 calories a day if half of those calories are from fat. When you realize that 42 percent, versus the suggested 15 to 20 percent, of the average American diet is from fat, it is little surprise that so many people are overweight. We really should not eat foods containing more than 10 percent fat. This adds a few more foods to the "watch it" list. Bacon is 94 percent fat, in addition to being a processed meat. Peanut butter is 75 percent fat. Palm oil and coconut oil are very high in saturated fat, although many food manufacturers are extracting them from their products as fast as they can, because of their bad reputations. But keep your eyes open for them, especially in snack items, granolas, and commercial cereals.

How about butter and margarine? *Both* (yes, margarine, too) contain 100 percent fat. Butter is high in cholesterol and saturated fat. And while margarine can boast of being cholesterol-free, health food it ain't—you are still eating *fat*. "But," you may argue, "it's polyunsaturated fat (versus saturated)." You may now know that polyunsaturated fats have their own horror story. They can lower desirable HDL levels and suppress the immune system. Their unstable molecular structure also tends to produce more oxygen-free radicals, which promotes rancidity and makes them carcinogenic (cancer-causing).

There's more. Part of the oil in margarine is hydrogenated (artificially *saturated*), a process involving high temperatures that makes an oil solid and spreadable. The bad news is that hydrogenation produces *trans fatty acids*, new dietary villains, which our bodies cannot process properly. Trans fatty acids raise triglyceride and cholesterol levels, and unfortunately constitute anywhere from 10 percent to 48 percent of margarine's total content. The softer the margarine, the fewer trans fatty acids. If margarine is a must in your life, try the squeeze-bottle brands.

At this point you're thinking that the butter/margarine choice is kind of like that kid's game "Would you rather burn to death or drown?", except that you have to decide between heart disease (butter) and cancer (margarine). How about neither? It's a small price to pay for living longer. But never fear, in lieu of abstinence, the next best word is moderation. A fair number of those I studied use butter and/or margarine and are perfectly healthy. However, a larger number of them use neither. They enjoy their toast dry or with an all-fruit jam, and they tell the waiters in the executive dining room to hold the mayo on their turkey sandwiches. One high-powered individual told me he decided to eliminate butter for one month so he could drop a few pounds. After losing the weight, he surprised himself by never returning to his days of "butter-filled English muffin crevices." He just doesn't miss the butter—nor the weight, which has stayed off for five years.

What oils can you consume without fearing for your life? Once again, I suggest: How about none? Use the evolutionary approach described in this book and try some of the recipes. It's possible, and it can be painless, I promise, to live without oils. But in the meantime (or during the weaning process), choose monounsaturated oils. These are oils such as canola oil, olive oil, peanut oil, and walnut oil. Canola oil is perhaps the best of all. It has the lowest saturated fat content, resists rancidity very well, has a low smoking point and is also delicious (it has a light taste). Olive oil is also good. It is the highest in monounsaturated fat. Many of the people I studied specifically mentioned using olive oil, including Arco's Camron Cooper, Eileen Ford, and Boeing's Malcolm Stamper. If you must have a butter-type topping on your bread, try lightly brushing it with olive oil—or ghee. Ghee is purified butter with no milk fat solids. It's perfect for those allergic to milk products. It can be heated to higher temperatures than butter without burning or getting rancid. By the way, never reuse any oil once it's been heated, since heating and/or storing oil increases the chances of its going rancid. (Another reason not to eat those fast-food French fries—or any fried food.) Also, keep oil refrigerated. The cold slows down the rancidity process by a third.

Keep in mind that all fats and oils contain varying percentages of saturated, polyunsaturated, and monounsaturated fats, but that all three are fats. And remember: *no* fat or oil is good for you.

So how do you cut down on fats besides reducing the obvious? Check a few labels and you'll catch on fast. You may like to try the following formula on a few foods to give you a better idea of where fats are waiting in ambush. To calculate the percentage of fat calories in a food, multiply the grams of fat in each serving (listed on the label) by 9. Then divide this number by the calories in each serving. Then multiply that by 100 and you get the total percent of fat calories in the food.

EXAMPLE: 2% LOWFAT MILK

$$1 \text{ cup } = 125 \text{ calories}$$
$$1 \text{ cup } = 5 \text{ grams of fat}$$
$$5 \text{ grams fat } \times 9 \text{ calories } = 45 \text{ calories of fat}$$
$$45/125 = 0.36$$
$$0.36 \times 100 = 36\% \text{ fat.}$$

(2% Lowfat milk is actually 36 percent fat.)

A CRASH COURSE ON CHOLESTEROL

It's time now for a few words about cholesterol. Cholesterol has had more media coverage than most celebrities. But, in spite of all the media hype, it can still be a complicated subject—so here's a crash course.

Your body needs cholesterol to produce hormones and construct cells. The liver produces more than 1,000 mg. of cholesterol a day and also filters and eliminates excess cholesterol. If the liver cannot do its job properly because there is too much cholesterol in the system or because it is genetically inadequate, excess cholesterol builds up on the walls of veins and arteries, clogging them and increasing the risk of heart disease. You want your total cholesterol number to be low and your HDL (high density lipoproteins) number to be high, since this is the enzyme that removes cholesterol from the system. The HDL average for adult Americans is 45 to 65, but it should be above 70 to protect against coronary artery disease. The ratio of total cholesterol to HDL is said to be the single best predictor of heart attack risk. Divide your total cholesterol by your HDL: the higher the figure, the greater the risk of developing heart disease. Dr. William Castelli, director of the Framingham Heart Study, says the ideal ratio is under 3.5 to 1. Anyone whose ratio is above 4.5 to 1 (4.5:1) should be treated to lower that ratio. Thus, a person with a supposedly "safe" total cholesterol level of 190 but a HDL level of only 35 has an *un*safe ratio of 5.4 to 1. The average victim of heart disease has ratios between 4.6:1 to 6.4:1 for women and 5.4:1 to 6.1:1 for men. In contrast, vegetarians have a low 2.8:1 ratio.

Cholesterol-reduction trials are shown to lower cholesterol a seemingly unimpressive 6.7 percent to 10 percent. By lowering your cholesterol just 10 percent, however, you reduce your risk of coronary heart disease by 30 percent. Every 1 percent drop in cholesterol in a person with high levels reduces the chances of developing heart disease by 3 percent. Every point you drop is important.

Exercise positively affects HDL, and food positively—or negatively—affects total cholesterol. But make sure you know where your cholesterol comes from. Only a third of blood pollutants are from the cholesterol we eat—the rest come from saturated fat. However, it is still prudent to keep a check on cholesterol intake. It is said that to maintain total cholesterol below 200 mg., we should eat no more than 300 mg. of cholesterol a day. Unfortunately, the average man consumes 500 mg. a day, and the average woman consumes 320 mg. Know your scores and don't kid yourself. If ratios confuse you, a simpler total cholesterol guide recommended by the National Cholesterol Education Program might offer some guidance. Since LDL (low density lipoproteins) are considered a separate risk factor for coronary heart disease, I list those guidelines as well.

	Total Cholesterol Guideline	LDL Guideline
Desirable	under 200	Below 130
Borderline-high	200–239	130–159
High	240 or more	160 or more

Note: 50 percent of Americans have borderline-high to high cholesterol levels.

Don't assume your cholesterol is low simply because you eat right and/or exercise. Dr. Bob Boni, CEO emeritus of Armco, is an avid exerciser but has a tendency toward high cholesterol. So, a few years ago he decided to educate himself on dietary cholesterol and make the appropriate changes. "I'm more cognizant of the necessity of low fat in the diet now," he says. "And I've lowered my cholesterol."

Unbelievably, all 20 year olds are said to already have some narrowing of the arteries. The worst news? *No symptoms are felt until arteries are 90 to 100 percent blocked*! Have your cholesterol levels tested regularly. A cholesterol test is considered the best prediagnosis for cardiovascular disease. It is said to be 85 percent accurate in diagnosis. Be sure to ask for an HDL blood test, as well. An HDL level below 35 is also considered a separate risk factor for heart disease. Also, keep your weight down. Every two pounds of excess weight adds 1 mg. to your total cholesterol.

If your total cholesterol is too high or your HDL is too low, you should exercise more, restrict eating animal products (the only place cholesterol is found, but more important, it is where saturated fats are found), eat more fish, and make sure you get enough vitamin E, lecithin, niacin, and calcium. Also, eat more soluble fiber.

Triglycerides are another type of blood fat associated with heart disease, particularly in women. The dietary culprits are rich foods, sugar, alcohol, and refined starches. Desirable levels fall between 30 to 150 mg. Dr. Castelli explains that triglycerides are part of a new high-risk picture for cardiovascular heart disease. Specifically, the danger signs are elevated triglyceride levels (160–220) and low HDL levels (usually under 40). He says this newly discovered high-risk group constitutes as much as 30 to 50 percent of those with heart disease.

VITAMINS: A WORTHY INVESTMENT?

So how do you know if your diet is giving you all you need? As with everything in life, balance is the key. The eating habits of the HWW leaders show that most eat a well-balanced diet containing daily servings of fruits, vegetables, grains, fish or meat, and dairy products. By following the basic executive diet outlined in the HWW Program, you will be on safe ground. Since the people I studied must, for the most part, however, restrict their daily calories, more than half take vitamin supplements as a backup. While they don't claim to be vitamin experts, they are well aware that missing vitamins and minerals can make them sluggish, hungry, and unproductive.

If you change your diet, you may be wondering if you're going to get all your nutrients without taking supplements. It depends. Your environment and lifestyle must be considered, since they can deplete vitamins from your system. Fluorescent lighting, for instance, depletes vitamin A. Alcohol and tobacco deplete potassium and vitamin C. Vitamins E and C, on the other hand, can help counteract the effects of city smog. Additionally, many foods are grown on "tired out" soil—soil that is depleted of vitamins and minerals because of overuse. Such soil produces food that looks normal but is not nutritionally "complete." Certainly you should aim to ingest the proper nutrients in your diet, but take a good multi-vitamin to be sure. If you are restricting your calories, take vitamins B and C. Vitamin B supplements vitamin and hormone deficiencies that may be distorting your appetite, and vitamin C can help block food cravings that are often brought on by mild allergic reactions.

If you want maximum nutrients for your calories, keep your food whole and basic, with minimal cooking and processing. The refining process robs many foods of essential nutrients. And steer clear of so-called "enriched" foods, which generally are poor in nutrients. "Enriched" white flour processing, for instance, takes out twenty nutrients and replaces only four. (The label should more accurately read "Sort of enriched," but I guess that wouldn't make a strong sales pitch.)

While I repeat that you needn't be a mathematician to eat correctly, the following charts may help you maintain an overview of the correct dietary balance.

Suggested Percentages of Total Caloric Intake*

Protein	15–20%
Carbohydrates	60–70 (Fiber—20–25 grams, not to exceed 35 grams)
Fat	15–25%

*Percentages fall somewhere between the most liberal and the most stringent suggested by experts in the field.

How close do we come to these percentages? On average, we consume only 45 percent carbohydrates—and *half* of that is from simple sugars. The Chinese eat 77 percent *complex* carbohydrates (unrefined). We also consume 42 percent fat—twice as much as we need. And just a word about sodium. While it is recommended by the National Academy of Sciences that we consume only 1,800 mg. a day, we in fact take in 3,000 to 4,000 mg. (two teaspoonfuls).

WHEN YOU EAT IS AS IMPORTANT AS WHAT YOU EAT

Breakfast: Eat It.   Very few of the men and women I studied skip breakfast (7 percent), but nearly 25 percent of all Americans miss this most important meal of the day. Studies show that people who miss breakfast eat at least as many calories as the rest of us (they make up for it later in the day when calories count even more) and, not surprisingly, they weigh more. Breakfast skippers have been found to consume more fat and cholesterol than breakfast eaters. Another plus: eating breakfast actually increases your metabolic rate (calories burned) by 10 percent.

Breakfast can be small, but be sure it is power-packed nutritionally. A high-fiber, sugarless whole-grain cereal (with nonfat milk) is the way most of these leaders get going, sustain a level amount of energy, and control their hunger until lunch. Unrefined complex carbohydrates (such as whole-grain breads and cereals) also boost your metabolic rate by as much as 10 percent for several hours, increasing both your energy level and the number of calories you burn. High-fiber foods give you more bulk with fewer calories, so you get full but not fat.

As with every aspect of the HWW Program, you must learn to tune in to your body and gear your choices accordingly. The best breakfast for one person may not necessarily work for another, although both may have identical lifestyles. Pay attention to your needs and treat yourself as you would a prized race horse. The proper nutritional combination in the morning will do more for you than a cup of coffee ever will.

Lunch: Watch for Hidden Calories. Nearly all the people in my study eat lunch (99 percent), while 23 percent of other Americans skip this midday boost. The standard executive lunch consists of salad (the number-one choice), a sandwich (tuna or turkey, without mayo, are favorites), or a noncreamy soup. If you're watching your weight, remember that people who have soup with a meal consume an average of 5 percent fewer calories and are just as satisfied.

Lunch is an excellent place to get in your protein for the day, and fish is an excellent choice. (Only 10 percent of the executives I studied mentioned having red meat for lunch.) But keep lunch light, since a heavy lunch can lower blood sugar, leading to midafternoon blahs (and the accompanying craving for something sweet). Currently, one-fourth of all meals in this country are eaten away from home, with lunch the overwhelming leader. If you eat lunch out, avoid fastfood restaurants. They currently capture half of the American restaurant dollar, but generally offer very little nutritional value for the money. Changes are being made toward more healthful menus, but fast foods are geared to please the palate rather than the body, with higher fat (30 percent), more sugar (50 percent), and more salt (60 percent) than the average American meal (which isn't a great standard to begin with). "Restaurants have a secret desire to kill people off," kids Bob Boni of Armco. They know Bob well at his favorite lunch haunt, because he always has the same thing—turkey on whole wheat with tomato, mustard, "and no mayo."

Several told me that their company cafeterias have become health-oriented in recent years, offering salad bars, lite-and-easy menus, or low-cholesterol selections. Randy Barron, president of Southwestern Bell, used to have biscuits and gravy for breakfast in the company cafeteria until the company changed its menu. Now he has a bran muffin, V8 juice, and decaffeinated coffee, and is not complaining—nor are his arteries. "I'm convinced you should eat your meals at the same time every day," adds Barron, who usually has a salad or soup for lunch. This is a good suggestion, since the body thrives on a consistent schedule. Regular feedings help your digestion and energy level and therefore help reduce hunger-induced binges.

A few of the people I spoke with brown-bag it, but most rely on the company cafeteria or a restaurant. Brown bagging can make meals a nutritional "plus," since bringing your lunch gives you more control over what you eat and when you eat it. Brown bagging also can save you time, calories, nutrition, and money. I know one busy business owner who pays someone to deliver her custom-made nutrition-packed "brown bag" every day, rather than order in from nearby gourmet restaurants. By the way, if you find carrying a brown bag humiliating, "briefcase" it. And even if you don't pack a lunch, you should have a few emergency semi-nonperishable snacks (such as apples, raw almonds, or rice cakes) stashed in your desk, briefcase or car. This circumvents the "Sure, I had a candy bar—I had to eat *some*thing!" excuse when you have to eat on the run. The HWW Diet & Nutrition Program will give you some brown bag tips later in the book.

Dinner: Light Is Right.   All of the HWW men and women eat dinner, though some nibble or eat lightly. For instance, USA Network's Kay Koplovitz says she just "grazes." If you are dieting and feel you absolutely must skip a meal, make it dinner. (However, don't nibble your way through the night on cookies and chips, call it "skipping dinner," and then complain about the scale not budging.) Claude Brinegar of Union Oil found he needed to drop a few pounds after a health scare. What worked best for him was cutting down on dinner. Dinner for Claude now might simply consist of an English muffin with low-fat cottage cheese—and he stays in great shape.

America's leaders eat *early*, and chicken is a big favorite. They also eat vegetables with (or *as*) dinner. Marcia Israel, founder of Judy's, likes "a heaping plate of every steamed vegetable I can think of . . . every color, so it's gorgeous and a foot high."

To Snack or Not to Snack.   What about snacking? Almost half—44 percent—of these leaders snack, but the majority of the snackers are at ideal weight. Snacking usually gets a bad rap. However, the *New England Journal of Medicine* reported that frequent nibbling may actually be better for a person's cholesterol level than three square meals a day. This is thought to be caused by the steady level of insulin that snacking maintains, which also accounts for a more constant blood sugar level. Steady blood sugar levels can help offset crazed hunger binges and are particularly good for those with hypoglycemia (low blood sugar). Nevertheless, if you choose to include snacking in your personal program, make sure not to use the "snacking is good for you" motto as a license to eat all day long. Also, be sure that the snacks you choose are nutritionally and calorically worthy of entering your "prized race horse" system.

Health convert and former sweet snacker Frederick Rentschler (Beatrice Co.) reports, "Sara (Lee) and Debbi (Fields) used to appear in my refrigerator all the time." He now curtails his sweet tooth and "sees Debbi" only on occasion.

The favorite snack of the people I interviewed is fruit, and the most popular snacking time is between 8 and 10 in the morning. "I try not to keep anything snacky in the house," says Eileen Ford of Ford Models, who limits her eating to three meals a day. Most agree that the best way to avoid temptation is to keep only healthful foods, such as fruit, in the house. Once again, it is a matter of your individual metabolism and finding what works best for *you*.

ALCOHOL, NICOTINE, AND CAFFEINE: LEGAL BUT LETHAL

Americans have many deeply ingrained, unhealthful habits, and alcohol, nicotine, and caffeine head the list. More than *one third* of the adult population is addicted to cigarettes, drugs, or alcohol. Half a million deaths a year are attributed to addictive diseases. Many of us begin using these substances at a tender age, usually in our teens, because we want to seem more adult. They are promoted through advertising, heavily factored in political lobbying, and generate a great deal of revenue.

If you are a regular user of any one of these substances, you are probably addicted. True, there are degrees and stages, but be aware and be honest with yourself in this area. While thinking of yourself as *an addict* might seem a bit overly dramatic or even painful, it is something you should confront. It could save your life and present an opportunity for growth that will make you stronger and more successful in everything else you do. Addictive substances lower our self-esteem along with our level of consciousness, since their purpose is to numb out reality, which pulls us away from our true nature. As former alcohol addict Ringo Starr described his new-found sobriety: "The difference is—I'm alive now!"

Here is an interesting stress-related fact: At least one study has shown that those best at handling stress also consume the least amount of alcohol, nicotine, and caffeine.

Alcohol, nicotine, and caffeine are bad for your health, period. The individuals I studied do not abuse these substances, and a significant number do not use them at all. Rather than preach, let me simply mention a few facts. You can figure it out from there.

Alcohol: "Just One" Can Hurt.   About 100 million Americans drink, and one out of ten is a problem drinker. In contrast, nearly 50 percent of the females and 14 percent of the males I studied are totally abstinent. Many drink only occasionally and few have more than two drinks a day or anything stronger than wine. Many have found that alcohol is directly related to weight gain, especially on the road. "The thing to really stay away from is alcohol," says LTV's Emmett Smith. "It lowers your resistance to food." Alcohol can also add pounds all by itself. Two cans of beer daily can add 33 pounds in one year. One glass of wine a day can add 10 pounds. But calories aren't the only reason alcohol makes you heavy. *Alcohol also inhibits your body's ability to burn fat by about a third* (per 3 ounces ingested). If the appeal to health and better living doesn't capture your attention, perhaps having a thinner waistline will.

At least one study has demonstrated that reducing alcohol is more important than reducing sodium in lowering blood pressure. Just one drink a day raises the risk of oral cancer by 60 percent. One drink a day also doubles the risk of breast cancer in women, and one drink a day can cause a decline in your ability to reason abstractly (synthesize new ideas), which is analogous to prematurely aging two to four years. Alcohol is, in the words of Nobel physicist Albert Einstein, "a poison." It kills brain cells, even in small doses. Over a period of time, two drinks a day can "age" your brain five to eight years. Drinking alcohol, even moderately, also contributes to memory loss. If you're looking for a "high," try exercise. Many say it gives that 5 o'clock cocktail pretty tough competition.

Nicotine: Sending Your Life up in Smoke.   Smoking is the #1 preventable cause of death in America today. Smoking kills more Americans *each year* than died in battle in World War II and Vietnam together. Sixty million Americans smoke—about one in four adults. Why do so many seem to ignore overwhelming medical statistics? One reason may be that cigarettes have the largest advertising budget of any consumer product, so people are literally being brainwashed.

Eighty-seven percent of the males and 90 percent of the females in my study do not smoke. However, many have had to kick the habit; they started smoking in their teens or twenties and then quit when the facts started to come in. Many experts have said that of all addictions, smoking is the hardest to kick. This is understandable, since smoking is now thought to raise endorphin levels, giving you the addictive runner's high feeling (and leaving you wanting more). Hard as it is to quit, many HWW leaders have done it. How did they do it? With persistence, determination, and commitment—the same principles that keep them exercising, eating right, and successful. The message? You can do it, too.

Want some moral support? Chevron's vice chairman, James Sullivan, quit smoking seven years ago, along with Chevron's CEO Ken Derr. They were going through a stressful situation during the merger of Gulf and Chevron and decided they wanted to eliminate at least one stressor: smoking. They signed up with Smoke Enders, and it worked. James jokes that it worked partly because "they make it so difficult for you to smoke with rules and record-keeping that you're ready to quit by your goal date" (twenty days for them). Chevron now offers the program free to employees and their families.

Redken's founder and CEO, Paula Kent Meehan, wasn't so lucky on her first few attempts. One time she was sure she had smoking beat and decided she could handle just "one or two" on a business trip to Japan. She handled one or two—and a lot more for several years. She recently quit for the last time and has some advice: "Once you've stopped, don't even have one—ever!"

Smoking accounts for an eye-opening 1,000 deaths a day in America. Half of all the heart attacks in women are a direct result of smoking. Smokers die at nine times the rate of nonsmokers. Even if you gained 20 percent of your weight after quitting, you'd still cut your risk of death in half. Cigarettes deplete vitamin C; one cigarette consumes 25 mg. of vitamin C. Finally, every cigarette raises total cholesterol half a percent on average, according to the American Health Foundation. The good news: cholesterol levels drop when you drop the cigarettes, and your lung tissue can repair itself.

Another tip for quitting is to get involved with an exercise program that you enjoy. Several told me that they became so wrapped up in their exercise habit that they were motivated to quit smoking so they could improve their performance. I believe them—I have seen this happen with more than one participant in my program at MCA/Universal. You might try it; it certainly can't hurt. Try anything, including professional help, if necessary. Most insurance plans now cover smokers' clinics. The bottom line is that smoking is *out* in the movies, *out* socially, and *out* in the corporate world. Many corporations are now smokefree, and the trend is expanding.

Caffeine: Not a HealthStyle "Plus".   Forty-five percent of the HWW leaders, male and female, do not drink coffee at all. Two or more cups of coffee a day is said to cause higher levels of stress. (Some of my clients even report that decaf can exacerbate their stress.) Coffee drinkers who have more than five cups a day are three times more likely to contract heart disease as are nondrinkers. Unfortunately, 20 percent of Americans drink five or more cups a day. Caffeine depletes calcium, decreases blood flow to the brain, and decreases Vitamin B absorption. It has been linked to lowered fertility in men, breast tumors in women, birth defects, elevated blood pressure, and ulcers.

Here is a listing of typical amounts of caffeine in most drinks:

Drip coffee	115 mg
Instant coffee	65 mg
Decaf coffee	2 mg
Tea	40 mg
Cola	10–25 mg

A client was once trying to con me into agreeing with the harmlessness of his few cups of coffee a day. What I finally said was, "The best I can say about coffee is that while a little may or may not hurt you, it definitely is *not* a HealthStyle 'plus,' so why do it? Why play with it?" Try to curtail your caffeine intake over a comfortable period of time. Start with cutting your levels in half, adjust to your new habit, and repeat this process at comfortable intervals until caffeine is at most a minimal part of your daily intake.

MAKE YOURSELF AN EXPERT ON YOU

Lest you tire of hearing how flawlessly wonderful these people are, I want to remind you once again that you can have what they have—what they have is "learnable." As busy as they are, the leaders in this book have made it a priority to acquire far more nutritional knowledge than the general population. The majority were even able to quote me their latest blood pressure and cholesterol scores. And they not only knew *what* they had eaten for breakfast, but they knew *why* they had eaten it. Invest a little time in educating yourself about nutrition. Start by subscribing to a quality magazine such as *American Health* or a health newsletter such as *Tufts University Diet & Nutrition Letter*. Read an occasional book on specific topics that pertain to you (such as arthritis or high cholesterol). One of the best, easy-to-read, unslanted, factual and entertaining (yes!) books on overall diet and nutrition is *Diet & Nutrition: A Holistic Approach* by Rudolph Ballentine, M.D. It's a great reference book to have on hand.

And while you may not be quite ready to take a class in nutrition, there are many excellent nutrition-oriented cookbooks available. "There are many good cookbooks and I'm always looking for more," says Janet Boni, the wife of Bob Boni of Armco, who formerly based nearly every main dinner course on cheese. Mrs. Boni recommends *Jane Brody's Good Food Book*.

Start making yourself an expert on yourself and the food you eat. Learn about wholesome foods and how to prepare them. Without doubt, it will be one of the wisest investments you've ever made, and you'll have fun doing it, too.

8 "BOTTOM LINE" NUTRITION TIPS:

1. Don't skip meals, especially breakfast.
2. Eat dinner early.
3. Eat fish two to five times a week. (Tuna counts, but skip the mayo.)
4. Snacking is okay, but make it healthful: fruit, rice cakes.
5. Limit red meat consumption to no more than once a week.
6. Avoid sugar, sugar substitutes, salt, caffeine, alcohol, cigarettes.
7. Avoid saturated and unsaturated fats. Use monounsaturated oils.
8. Eat lots of fruits and vegetables.

TIPS TO REMEMBER

- *The HWW successes have better health and eating habits than the average American.*
- *They see a little weight gain as a red flag and do something about it.*
- *Their favorite food is fish—which other Americans seldom eat.*
- *They eat more salads and cereal than other Americans.*
- *They rarely eat desserts.*
- *They consume less sugar, fat, salt, and red meat than other Americans.*
- *Know your cholesterol, HDL, and blood pressure scores.*
- *87 percent of the HWW men and 90 percent of the HWW women do not smoke. 14 percent of the men and 40 percent of the women do not drink alcohol. 25 percent do not drink coffee.*

Special Tip: Add powdered vitamin C to your water bottle and keep it on your desk.

ENJOY THE PROCESS

Chapter Four

EXERCISE AND SUCCESS

TIPS FROM THE TOP

The fitness craze of the Eighties is now the gospel. Exercise is the best free lunch in town.

— *Charles Kittrel, Phillips Petroleum*

WHY EXERCISING LIKE "EVERYBODY ELSE" CAN MAKE YOU GAIN WEIGHT

The fact is, when it comes to keeping our bodies healthy, Americans are not doing much better than they are with their mental fitness (see Chapter Seven). Americans suffer from the highest rate of degenerative diseases in the world. One reason for this may be that a large percentage of us really don't exercise. Only 54 percent of us claim we exercise regularly, compared to 76 percent of the HWW men and women. More factually, the Centers for Disease Control report that *a surprisingly low 8.2 percent of us exercise at a frequency, duration, and intensity considered desirable for good health,* according to the now standard government recommendation (some form of exercise vigorous enough to elevate breathing and heart rates but not so vigorous that it becomes impossible to talk comfortably—fifteen to twenty-five minutes, three to four times a week). While the CDC reported another 34 percent of American adults were "regularly active," it was found that their exercise regimes did not meet the government rec-ommendation. The discrepancy between this and other studies is thought to be due to the fact that people tend to overestimate the time they spend exercising. Also, the CDC surveys asked precise questions with detailed definitions while most studies leave terms like "regular exercise" to the discretion of the participants. The point: people probably are not exercising as much as they think they are.

Not *one* person in my study labeled himself inactive, while, CDC findings aside, a startling 41 percent of us label ourselves as "not active." The HWW leaders have been exercising an average of eighteen years, while 25 percent of Americans who do exercise have just begun within the last year (and over half will quit within the first six months). Instead of exercising, too many come home from work at night and plop down on the couch for America's favorite recreational activity—watching TV, which we do for an average of seven hours a day. It is said that children spend more time watching TV than they spend in school on a yearly basis! Worse, this nationally popular form of "relaxation" can no longer even be viewed as a legitimate excuse for being a couch potato. According to a recent survey, watching two or more hours of TV can actually contribute to your anxiety level instead of reducing it! Further, studies show that children watching two or more hours of TV a day are twice as likely to have high cholesterol (over 200). Four or more hours a day increases the likelihood to four times. Since 175 is considered a high cholesterol level for any child over age two, these statistics become even more unfortunate. It seems that heavy TV viewers are more fearful and suspicious of strangers. They also buy more guns, watchdogs, and elaborate home security systems.

Our favorite exercise is walking, compared with tennis and running, the more active favorites of the HWW leaders. While walking is justifiably the safest and most enduring form of exercise to date, some experts have once again questioned the accuracy of the public's actual participation in walking as exercise. When filling out an intimidating exercise questionnaire, it is easier to be more careless on walking estimates than tennis or running, for example. Those repeated trips to the coffee machine can suddenly become "regular daily walking" when pen goes to paper. However, even if we really do walk as much as we say we do, it is interesting to note that these leaders as a group choose more rigorous forms of exercise. They apparently approach their workouts as intensely as their careers. They also manage to stick to their regimes better than most other Americans, even though 60 percent travel more than ten weeks a year.

Of those in my study who exercise regularly, a large number were athletes in high school or college. In fact, Charles Kittrel wagered during one of our talks that a high percentage of successful executives were "former jocks." He was right! One example. Former Westinghouse CEO, John Marous, is a "real" athlete. He played semi-pro baseball before and during his beginning years at Westinghouse (while simultaneously getting his Master's degree). In fact, had it not been for an arm injury, John may have gone on to play serious ball and never have become CEO and chairman of Westinghouse. In one instance John helped pull his team out of financial difficulties, and ended up being owner, manager, and infielder at the same time. And when Westinghouse transferred him at one point, John wasted no time in establishing a bowling league as well as organizing a Westinghouse team in a softball league—and winning trophies!

SUCCESS MAXIM: BRAWN BREEDS BRAIN

While many of those I talked to must watch their diets continually, most of these same men and women say that exercise comes a lot more naturally. They love to exercise and are rightfully proud of their fitness achievements.

They also are true believers when it comes to the benefits of exercise. "I need my morning walk. It's my cup of coffee—and my dogs love it!" says Camron Cooper of Atlantic Richfield, who goes to the beach for her dawn walks. Charles Kittrel sums up nicely the exercise philosophy of those at the top: "What sense does it make for people to spend years improving their minds, only to have their bodies collapse prematurely or function inefficiently?"

The important thing to remember is this: Nearly every leader I studied who exercises regularly is within his or her ideal weight range. Think about this, because it's a simple answer to a big problem facing 77 percent of the American public today. If you want to control your weight, you will improve your odds if you exercise. It's a simple fact.

But exercise and physical fitness do a lot more than help control your weight. Physical fitness also teaches us mental success. It's like learning to play the piano. Once you learn to play the scales, you can use them to play waltzes, jazz, or rock. Accordingly, the habit of physical fitness (that is, physical "success") is translated to every aspect of one's life, including mental fitness. In the words of Paul Oreffice, the head of Dow Chemical, "I truly believe that if the body is in good shape, the mind is in better shape. I notice the correlation." There is something to be said for the relationship between sheer physical strength and mental strength, and that is this: Changes in the body take place at the same rate in the mind. In other words, there is a direct correlation between handling physical demands and handling life's demands. Specifically, exercise establishes the qualities of persistence, stamina, integrity, and risk-taking, such as pushing beyond your personal limits. (An extra bonus: when physical energy is released, mental and creative energies are liberated as well, according to experts.) The HWW leaders I interviewed are perfect examples of the "Brawn Breeds Brain" maxim—most were physically "successful" (fit) before they reached the top. They developed the habit of success *before* they became successful.

Instead of being held back by your own doubts and fears when you are facing a career challenge or would like to make a life change, you can find that exercise promotes a positive attitude that says, "If I can do this, anything is possible."

How Exercise Improves Your Performance

- Workers who exercise produce 2 to 5 percent more output than nonexercisers.
- Exercise raises deep body temperature, causing a rise in alertness and performance for several hours.
- Exercisers are less tired, more disciplined, more relaxed, and more productive at work. They have increased confidence and concentration, a better self-image, and more optimism and energy.
- Memory tests show 20 percent improvement by increasing oxygen to the brain with exercise.
- Absenteeism is reduced by as much as 42 percent through regular exercise.
- Reaction times of physically active older men (average age 56) are 20 percent faster than the reaction times of sedentary men.
- Exercise releases aggression and lowers tension. The less active have a 52 percent greater chance of developing hypertension.
- Exercisers have fewer aches and pains (exercise-induced endorphins are natural painkillers).
- Nonexercisers are more likely to have sleep problems.

The conclusions you can draw from these statistics are obvious: Exercise can improve your work performance, and better work performance can increase your success in whatever you do. There's another payoff from exercise if you're involved in corporate sports and fitness activities: getting better acquainted with your associates and building up your contacts. It is no secret that people who work together often play together. You can play tennis, golf, run, cycle to work, or do other activities with your colleagues and participate in office sports events as well. One CEO, when applying for an upper-level position in his "early days," walked into his interview and recognized his would-be boss was a member of his cycling club. "It certainly broke the ice," he says, "and I got the job." Many of those in my study repeatedly emphasized the importance of having a mentor and getting along well with those around (and above) you. I notice the camaraderie at my MCA/Universal program. I often hear someone saying, "Oh, so *you're* [John Doe]! I've talked to you on the phone before, but I never knew what you looked like."

While a trimmer physique may not lead directly to a fatter paycheck or the CEO desk, remember that the people in this study got healthy (at average age 35) before they got wealthy (at average age 39). More important, they have proven by where they are today that getting healthy was one of the wisest investments they ever made.

NOT FUN, NOT DONE: CHOOSING THE RIGHT PROGRAM FOR YOU

The successes I studied participate in an astounding variety of physical activities. One runs 50-mile races; another has climbed Mount Everest twice. One enjoys whitewater rafting and rock climbing (even though her husband prefers to keep his feet on solid ground). One is a triathlete, one is an ultra-marathoner, four are marathoners, and another competes in downhill skiing. Many are excellent tennis or racquetball players, and others play a mean game of golf. Keep in mind that the average age of these corporate jocks is 55.

A fair percentage of those I studied do calisthenics, and at least half engage in walking—either as their sole form of exercise or, more commonly, in conjunction with their other workout routines.

Many have exercise equipment in their homes, and several are so dedicated that they have complete gyms. A gym is a nice "plus," but don't use it as an exercise loophole: "Ah-ha! I'll get with the program just as soon as I set up that gym. *That'll* do it!" Having the latest flashy high-tech equipment or sporting the trendiest designer workout labels will not hand you a new body on a silver platter. Too often, people who spend money on expensive exercise equipment find that it is just taking up space in the closet.

Although the buddy system can be a great motivation enhancer, Kathryn Klinger found coordinating schedules with her girl-friends too complicated and sticking with it alone too hard, so she opted for a professional trainer. Interestingly, Kathryn thanks the

New York City public school system for giving her a good aerobic conditioning background rather than a sports background. She thinks this is unusual; most school athletic programs favor competitive sports over life fitness sports. Charles Kittrel agrees. He thinks the public education system "pampers the gifted athlete." Kittrel believes schools should teach that fitness is for everyone. He points out that 60 percent of America's children are below average fitness levels for their age groups.

Kittrel advises those of you who are just starting an exercise program to not do too much too soon, and "Don't do the same thing all the time—it's boring and too hard on the body." The truth is, you should keep every aspect of your life stimulating and interesting. Dr. Bob Boni of Armco and his wife, Janet, do. For example, they will go to ballet for a period of time and then choose something else when the slightest hint of boredom creeps in. Don't be afraid to experiment with athletic activities, too. Just make sure you do *something* consistently.

Variety is important, but no more important than enjoying your workout. "Find something you enjoy," says Emmett Smith. "If you'd rather face death in the desert than exercise, you won't stay with it. It's a rare person who can do something that he really doesn't enjoy for the sake of his health." Kraft's Arthur Woelfle couldn't agree more and brings up an interesting point: "To have an active mind, you need an active body, but to exercise when it's a tremendous chore is worse for you" (body chemistry is negatively affected when you dislike what you do—which applies to your career as well). Colombe Nicholas couldn't agree more. This president emeritus of Christian Dior says her baby keeps her moving and she feels no embarrassment in not having a structured exercise program. In fact, she jokes, "We have an exercycle in the bathroom, and we couldn't do without it. We use it as a valet—my husband gets the handle bars and I get the seat" (alas, another "dust-collecting equipment" statistic). Likewise, Mary Kay of Mary Kay Cosmetics keeps moving at work but does not do formal exercise. "I'm president of Exercise Anonymous—call me if you feel like exercising and I'll talk you out of it." While many do work out at elite fitness levels, others don't and still stay in shape.

The once-popular fitness motto, "No pain, no gain," is fittingly replaced by the credo "Not fun, not done." You must find that special combination of time, place, and activity that spells fun for you. Do *whatever* you have to do to make your workouts as enjoyable as possible.

Later in this book, you will learn how to start with a specific routine and gradually customize it to your likes, needs, and schedule, just as the men and women in this book have done.

THE SECRET TO EXERCISE SUCCESS

The HWW HealthStyle is an attitude as much as a tangible program. Exercise is not viewed as a chore or something you think of getting out of with business emergencies. Instead, it represents an attitude that you *want* to move your body at every opportunity possible throughout the day. Cultivate this attitude and you will soon find creative ways to work exercise into your day, even when your regular workout is unavoidably sabotaged. Gilda Marx says, "I take every fitness opportunity all day long. I park far away, I take the stairs, I do stomach and dynamic tension exercises in the car."

The secret to exercise success is amazingly fundamental: *Move* it and *keep* moving it. The men and women move their bodies in any way possible throughout the day, to keep their blood moving, their metabolism up, and their minds alert. Dow Chemical's CEO, Paul Oreffice, follows these principles and so does his wife. He says, "She's in constant motion. She weighs less now than when we got married thirty-six years ago."

The American lifestyle has become more sedentary over the years. Think of the active life of the Pilgrims (or even your grandparents), who often used their bodies morning until night without stopping or complaining. We've all heard the "I walked five miles to school in the snow—barefoot" stories. Incorporate just a bit of that mentality. Visualize each movement as putting one more log on your metabolic (calorie-burning) fire. Your metabolic rate stays boosted for up to 24 hours after exercising, so that flight of stairs you opt for instead of taking the elevator represents more than a mere minute or two of exercise. Incidentally, for each pound of muscle you add through your workouts, you will burn 50 to 100 more calories each day.

Here's a story to help imprint the log-on-the-metabolic-fire concept. My father, an executive with a bad back, unknowingly helped inspire this book (for a number of reasons). He used to live year-round in Minnesota and, during the winter, kept a fire going in the evenings by descending the two flights of stairs to the basement and carrying up wood, one or two logs at a time. After observing this almost pitiful sight for a number of years, age introduced guilt to his five kids, and we finally offered to assume the loathsome log-carrying task (laziness and the fear of centipedes and basement monsters made this a heroic gesture). Strangely, Dad emphatically rejected our offers, insisting that this was his "back therapy." He said, "Just a little bit is all it takes! You get the blood pumping and miracles happen." Talk about reprogramming the mind and creating opportunities! Needless to say, we didn't want to deprive him of his "therapy."

Here's another "little bit" example: A secretary who exchanges her manual typewriter for an electric one, but keeps her diet and lifestyle otherwise the same, will gain four to six pounds a year. Another: just the act of standing up from a sitting position increases the heart rate (and thus metabolic rate) by 10 beats per minute, as well as increasing alertness. It doesn't take much to keep your metabolic fire stoked. (For some practical "little bit" ideas, see "Every Little Bit Helps," page 191).

HOW EXERCISE CHALLENGES BRING OUT THE COMPETITIVE EDGE

Interestingly, tennis is the number-one sport of the executives. Tennis is all about competition; it involves winning or losing. It perhaps is no surprise that a good portion of the HWW leaders, both male and female, admitted they enjoy triumphing over opponents. Others prefer competing with themselves by constantly improving their times or accomplishments in workouts, and there are those who are happiest not to compete at all. One CEO is an accomplished runner but refrains from racing, opting instead to "smell the roses," and enjoy his workouts without pressure.

Another corporate jock philosophizes: "Struggling against a worthy opponent brings out the best in us. It gives us a measure of our own performance, develops our self-confidence, and lets us reach new levels of potential."

Malcolm Stamper's (Boeing) wife received a gold medal in a NASTAR ski event several years ago at age 57, which has presented a challenge to Mal. So far he has won seven silvers and one bronze, but no gold. When he hired an instructor to help improve his technique, the first thing she said to him was "Your problem, Mr. Stamper, is that you're skiing out of control and not fast enough." She said, "If you want to go on skiing when you get older (Mal laughs, because he was 58 at the time), you're going to have to learn to ski better." Mal relates, "She then tore apart my whole technique and put me on Cybernetics (mental skills), which has changed things substantially." His comment on the subject now at the age of 66: "I'm going to get that gold medal now!"

WHY YOU SHOULD WALK—& HOW TO STAY WITH IT

Even though competitive activities may be your preference, consider walking as part of your routine. Walking is America's most popular exercise and can be ideal for weight maintenance and as part of your baseline conditioning (or Regular Recurrent Exercise, as described in the Exercise Program). A daily 30-minute walk can burn 18 pounds worth of calories in a year. Establishing the walking habit can be compared to establishing a water drinking habit in that they both seem *too* simple ("Nothing could be happening when it's this easy.") But give it a chance. The executives did, and now many are hooked.

Walking is a perfect noninjury exercise. It is also a great rehabilitator for injuries. Lucky Stores' Larry DelSanto used to jog, but quickly adapted to walking when his knees gave him trouble. He now keeps in shape by walking one to four miles four days a week and playing golf once or twice a week.

If you find walking boring, try walking to music, books on tape, walking (and talking) with a partner, or repeating a positive "mantra," (such as "I am capable of anything I choose to do"). Or bring along a small pad and pencil and jot down creative thoughts along the way. Also, try taking different routes. Redken's CEO, Paula Kent Meehan, says "While my husband exercises every day of his life very precisely—the same routine at the same time—I need variety. I take a different walking route every day."

"I've learned to walk stairs," says Marcia Israel, who deliberately chooses a high floor in the hotel when she's on the road. Incidentally, when Marcia "takes" the stairs, she isn't walking, she's *running*—and it's often twenty floors at a time! *Just walking up and down two flights of stairs a day can burn up to six pounds of calories in a year.* It is said that stair climbing expends more energy than jogging, swimming, cycling, or calisthenics. Marcia is a great example of someone who is not an avid fitness buff but who has made subtle changes in her lifestyle that add up to better health. She proves that an all-or-nothing attitude is not a requirement for fitness.

WHAT KEEPS THEM MOTIVATED CAN GET YOU GOING

"Staying in shape to do the things I want to do motivates me," says Charles Kittrel, who has semi-retired since our first interview and currently describes himself as a "ski bum." "It's my wife who motivates and inspires me," says Emmett Smith of LTV. His wife of forty-one years, Teresa, says: "Emmett has found his activity (running), and I have found mine (tennis), and we don't cross over. You have to like what you're doing." Feeling good motivates Teresa: "You know from experience that after you exercise it's a whole different world—and it doesn't cost any money!" Emmett also exercises to feel good, but jokes, "Running 35 miles a week gets you out of doing work around the house—my wife doesn't have the courage to ask me to mow the lawn." Emmett has run two ultra-marathons (50 miles) and says he was motivated to pursue running in 1976 when he ran in a 10K with running pros Bill Rogers and Frank Shorter. "I'll never forget it—they looked like they'd been shot out of a cannon. I never saw anyone move that fast." The experience made him want to try harder, and pretty soon "I was in the running scene." That's for sure! Emmett ran a marathon at age 60 and finished second in his age group. But most important, Emmett says, "I love the camaraderie of running. In your running shorts, everybody looks alike, more or less. Nobody knows what you do for a living."

What motivates Chevron's James Sullivan to stay fit? "I want to accomplish things and make a contribution. When I feel good about myself, look good and fit in my clothes, I feel I'm in control of myself and that gives me a much brighter, more positive outlook which impacts other people. I think people want to look up to you and say 'He has his act together and knows what's going on.' Feeling well, looking good and being mentally and physically alert are all part of that."

At 65, Dow Chemical's Paul Oreffice believes that keeping fit is like running a business. "You must always challenge the system," he says. Paul is motivated to continually improve his tennis game so he can beat his younger opponents.

"We've decided we're just not going to get old," says exercise advocate Marge Barron of herself and her husband Randy, president of Southwestern Bell. They take frequent walks together, and whenever the weather is bad, they drive to a local indoor mall to walk.

Paul Lego, CEO of Westinghouse, runs 30 pre-dawn miles a week because "It keeps me fit, burns off the stress, and gives me quiet time to think." Lego is 58, weighs 165 pounds, and runs five miles in less than an hour. Not one to waste time, Paul often solves business problems while running—as if a 60-hour work week weren't enough! But Lego is not a workaholic by definition. He never takes work home during the week or on weekends. Lego and his wife, Ann, are avid golfers and have been married 32 years.

The first motivational boost for exercise enthusiast John Teets, former CEO of Greyhound, came from his high school track coach. "He didn't allow smoking or soft drinks. He would throw you off the team if he caught you." (I hesitate to imagine what action he would have taken with alcohol and drugs.) "He was really ahead of his time in regard to sugar and caffeine. He influenced a lot of kids back then."

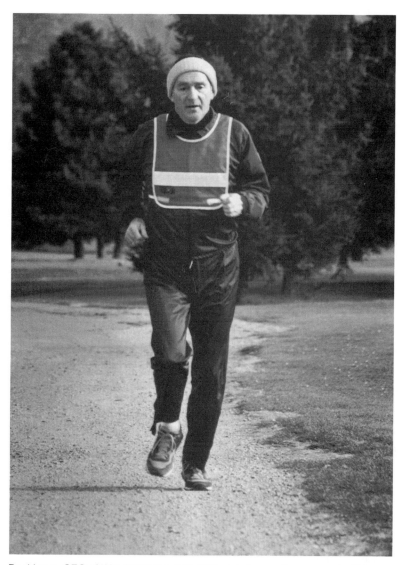

Paul Lego, CEO of Westinghouse, runs thirty pre-dawn miles per week. "It keeps me fit, burns off the stress, and gives me quiet time to think."

Teets was a high hurdler with four varsity letters. Another motivational boost for Teets came with a little different type of packaging later in life. A few years ago he fell through the ceiling while repairing his roof. He was hospitalized with a punctured lung, broken collar bone and pelvis, but within a month was beginning to move around—against his doctor's orders. His wife, equally fitness conscious, helped him to maneuver, his arm around her neck. "She literally almost dragged me around the neighborhood—a real pitiful sight, according to my incredulous neighbors. I was determined to get back."

High Energy Is a Big Motivator.   Survival seems to be what drove many of America's top leaders to discover fitness long before it became popular. They quickly figured out that they needed energy to survive—and succeed—in the fastpaced corporate world. They also realized that good health yields higher energy. Simple deductive reasoning told them to pursue good health and fitness for more energy and success. Robert Gilmore, who started as a machinist at Caterpillar Tractor fifty years ago and worked his way up to being president, says, "The successes are the hard workers, but you have to have lots of energy." Now, an avid skier at the age of 72, Gilmore is still going strong.

Five daughters have not slowed down Debbi Fields, who had her fourth baby on a Thursday and was back at work on Friday. She says, "I'm really a high energy person." Mary Kay (Cosmetics), who didn't start her business until she was middle-aged and retired, says, "I love my work and feed off the energy. I had five back-to-back meetings yesterday, but I felt more energized when I was done than when I began." Neither Debbi nor Mary Kay has a regimented exercise program, but both keep very physically active in their work.

Exercise, not caffeine, gives Gilda Marx, CEO of Gilda Marx Industries, a nice, even, high energy level. She says, "I'm not high strung, I'm high energy." She adds, "I don't have an age, just an energy level." (Gilda also believes that using your creative talent helps. She says, "Creativity turns on the energy.")

And finally, a little motivational insight from Conoco's Sam Schwartz. Sam is retired now and feeling better than ever. But he wishes he had been more motivated to exercise while he was working. "I am exercising more now that I've retired and I have more energy than ever. But I wish that I had built more exercise into my life when I was working—I would have had more energy. It's a dilemma—if you are tired and your job is demanding, you don't think you have the energy to exercise. Conversely, when you're exercising, you realize you can't do the job as well without exercising."

So, if a trimmer waistline and lower cholesterol level aren't powerful enough reasons to exercise, perhaps the promise of *more energy* will motivate you to get started.

HOW TO FIT FITNESS INTO A BUSY SCHEDULE

"Exercise is built into our family's lifestyle."
—Malcolm Stamper, Boeing

How do these busy leaders find time for exercise? Once again, they have managed to find solutions that work. "Running is very high on my priority list," says one CEO. "Last night, I could have gone to dinner with friends or to a basketball game, but I hadn't run that morning, so I ran last night."

Do you think it's too hard to get out of bed to exercise in the morning? Lyle Everingham, CEO of Kroger Co., does an hour of concentrated exercise (jogging and calisthenics) before the birds get up. He works out from 5:30 to 6:30 every morning like clockwork, then is ready to face the day. Philip Smith of General Foods combines stress management with his early morning workout—he runs, showers, then meditates. If these humans (the same species as you and I) can break a predawn sweat and still put in a full day running a major corporation and then get motivated—so can we!

Not surprisingly, most of the successes I spoke with are "scheduled exercisers," which is the example you want to follow. Too often it just doesn't happen if you "wait to see how the day goes." It appears that they are fairly evenly divided between morning and evening workouts. Most found their daily work schedules too unreliable to trust getting in a lunch-hour workout on a regular basis. They generally exercise immediately before or immediately after work. (See Chapter 6 for more help with finding time.)

EXERCISE AND TRAVEL: BE A ROAD RUNNER

The leaders in my study have had a lot of practice at fitting their workouts into their travels, and most are quite successful at it. Exercise can boost energy, regulate sleep, and combat jet lag when you're traveling. Richard Morrow of Amoco jogs in whatever city he's in, as does Rocky Johnson of GTE and James Evans of Union Pacific. It is no accident that Dow Chemical's Paul Oreffice has not missed one day of exercise on the road (or anywhere else) in eleven years! He has learned to modify his routine for the road: "I put a towel over the door and do my chin-ups. I can't carry my Nautilus board with me but I take my leg weights."

Southwestern Bell's Randy Barron has also had to resolve the travel problem, with his twenty weeks a year of travel. He says he tries to stay at hotels with workout facilities—"There are more and more of them these days." Or he will take advantage of the hotel pool, substituting swimming for his regular workout when he travels.

While hotels with exercise facilities are increasing, Robert McCowan of Ashland Oil says that you shouldn't rely on them. "Don't rely on equipment or you can lose the exercise habit easily." The lesson? Be committed, but be flexible. McCowan said that his calisthenics/running program is actually easier when he's on the road, because there are fewer distractions. Distractions or not, McCowan hasn't missed a workout in seven years.

Running or walking in a new city can be stimulating, and any good hotel should be able to recommend the good spots. Also, keep in mind that many health clubs now have temporary memberships available. It's probably even covered on your expense account. Sticking to your program in a new environment presents a challenge—something no winner worth his or her salt can resist.

TRY THE EXERCISE ELIXIR

"You need to succeed."

—Richard Morrow, CEO, CB emeritus, Amoco Oil

LTV's ultrarunner, Emmett Smith, says, "All I know is that I feel better mentally and physically when I exercise. If I don't do it, I feel out of sorts." Emmett was badly overweight in his thirties and did not exercise at all. He began twenty-two years ago when his company started an exercise program. When he got serious about running, he lost 30 pounds, and he has kept it off. He says he loves the "relaxed tiredness" he feels after running. Whenever you need a motivational boost, remember that the executives do their own sweating; they have had to work for their health—and their highs. Fitness is one thing that can't be subcontracted.

Exercise can serve you in many ways, psychologically as well as physiologically. It gives you energy if you are feeling down (by increasing oxygen), or it can act as a natural tranquilizer if you are strung just a little too tight. Observe yourself. Notice how you crave a snack, a drink, or a nap after work (or lunch). Just when you think you're too tired to blink, after putting in more than a full day, rejuvenate yourself with the exercise elixir. By choosing exercise, you may eliminate falling victim to those energy dips, and you can lose weight in the process.

TIPS
TO REMEMBER:

Consistency counts: the HWW leaders have exercised an average of 18 years; they were "fit first, successful second."

- *They are hooked on exercise, and enjoy improving their fitness skills. (Choose the right program. Enjoy the process.)*
- *Frequency helps adherence. Once or twice a week is not enough.*
- *Find ways to work exercise into your day.*
- *Keep up your exercise while traveling.*
- *Exercise reduces hunger and increases metabolism (burning of calories).*
- *Those who exercise regularly are within their ideal weight range.*
- *Exercise doesn't take your energy, it gives you energy.*

COMMIT

Chapter Five

PSYCHING UP FOR SUCCESS

TAKING CHARGE AND STAYING CHARGED

Staying physically fit is like keeping a corporation on track. The foundation is the vision of the desired future state of the corporation. Once the vision is defined, it is essential to focus all decisions and actions on achieving that state. Similarly, an individual has to envision that desired future physical/emotional state and focus personal decisions and actions on achieving it. I have that picture in my mind. The problem is to avoid the rationalization that certain actions will not sidetrack me.

—Bob Boni, CEO emeritus, Armco

A Motivation Quiz

Are you self-motivated? *Seventy percent of us know precisely how much exercise we need to stay healthy, and what kind of food to eat and how much. We just don't do it.* Why? Lack of motivation is a major factor. Are you one of those few people who are self-motivated? Before you answer, think about this question: What happened to last year's New Year's resolutions (or don't you bother making them anymore)? If you still aren't sure about your motivation level, take the following quiz.

1. When you begin a program, you usually:

    (a) Start with grand goals and do everything perfectly—for awhile.

    (b) Start on a whim, after reading a magazine program.

    (c) Start slowly and customize the program to suit your likes and needs.

2. If the phone rang just as you were leaving for the gym to exercise and the caller had a "now or never" offer to attend the concert of your dreams, you would:

    (a) Say Yes and cancel your workout.

    (b) Say Yes and do 15 minutes at home instead of going to the gym for your usual 60-minute workout.

    (c) Say No and do your full workout per your routine.

3. If brownies were being circulated at the office, you would:

    (a) Eat one and increase your workout later.

    (b) Resist and not feel deprived.

    (c) Resist and feel deprived.

SCORING:

1. (a) 0 points	(b) 0 points	(c) 2 points
2. (a) 0 points	(b) 2 points	(c) 1 point (too fanatical)
3. (a) 1 point	(b) 2 points	(c) 0 points

If you scored the maximum 6 points, you may need no further motivation. If not, a little "motivation therapy" may be in order. Read on!

THE BEST WAYS TO STAY MOTIVATED

The "Snap Factor."   The Snap Factor is that state of mind when you temporarily snap into a program, usually at the onset. It is the honeymoon—you are strong and do everything perfectly and effortlessly. Discipline is not an issue. But then, inevitably and insidiously, things start to slide, and you can't stop the fall. It is hope, adrenalin, a new toy, but it is *not* true motivation. True HealthStyle motivation intelligently sees you through the highs and lows, day in and day out, and is usually cultivated. However, if you understand the Snap Factor for what it is, you can identify it, capitalize on it, and be prepared with an alternative plan when it wears off.

Do You Really Want to Change?   Why bother with any of this "HealthStyle stuff" if things seem to be rolling along all right in your life? For one thing, good health habits can increase your life expectancy as much as thirteen years. And, as with most anything, *if you're not moving forward, you're moving backward.* Or, to paraphrase Bob Dylan, you're either being born or you're dying. Although almost everyone I interviewed claimed to be happy with his or her career status, their prevailing philosophy was that you must always strive to do better, to improve yourself—in fitness, career and life. One example: the muscle mass of the average American decreases by 10–12% between the ages of 30 and 65 (unless you *do* something about it). So, if you aren't taking positive steps forward, you are slowly and insidiously slipping backward. *There is no such thing as standing still.* Why "fix it if it ain't broke?" Because if you don't—it *will* break, sooner than later.

The successes I studied are doing a lot of things right that help them stay motivated, such as enjoying their food and exercise. Good for them, but how can you do it, too?

First, you must seriously *want* to change, not just lose a few pounds for Aunt Lulu's wedding next month. Webster says that motivation is "something within a person that incites him to action." It is something you want deep down—internally—that can be nurtured, not something that you can slap on at will. Remember that old joke: "How many psychiatrists does it take to change a light bulb? Only one, but the light bulb has to really *want* to change." But being motivated to change isn't the only factor. You must then have a substantive doable program that can help change the way you see yourself and *keep* you motivated along the way, which is the purpose of this book.

Studies say the single most important psychological obstacle to regular exercise and good diet is lack of motivation. How do we make ourselves do what we know we should do? Is it simply a matter of following a few common sense "basics," such as setting goals? My experience says no. While I'm happy to see a growing trend in more well-balanced programs and fewer fanatical fads, failure rates for all programs remain high. Common-sense basics alone aren't the answer. Nor are fear motives. Health-related statistics or even a personal health scare may move us to change our behavior for awhile, but it generally doesn't hold. I've found that staying motivated is also a matter of grasping the psycho-dynamics of how to break deeply ingrained patterns of behavior (habits) and how to establish new ones.

It's All About Habits.   Unfortunately, changing just one habit presents a big enough problem for most people. Changing several habits can seem overwhelming. The good news is that once you understand the generic formula for making and breaking habits, each individual habit no longer presents such a problem.

Habit Strategy.   The secret for making or breaking a habit is to first stay motivated long enough to secure a behavioral change. You can *decide* to quit smoking or lose weight, but that is only the conscious mind at work. The subconscious mind is much slower to change and needs more time to break a lifetime pattern. So how do you stay motivated long enough to let the new pattern "sink in" to the subconscious, to stabilize the habit? You can do this by applying the "Eleven Proven Steps to Motivation" that follow. We depend more on the external motivational factors such as goals, rewards, spouse support, and progress charts to keep us motivated in the beginning stages. But the internal factors enable us to eventually replace many of the external factors (such as rewards) by behavior that is intrinsically motivated. Being motivated then is no longer something you *seek* and nurture, it is something you *are*.

Once you get yourself going toward a new and improved HealthStyle, you need to keep yourself going. The following Eleven Proven Steps to Motivation are the keys to your new HealthStyle. Some have already been discussed; others are explained in this chapter. The first five steps are the External Steps, and they will help you with the logistical "how-to" day-to-day aspects. The remaining six are the Internal Steps, and they can equip you psychologically for the ups and downs of your HealthStyle program. I've refined them over many years of work and research, and I *know* they work. If you implement these steps into your diet, exercise, and stress management programs, you will become "motivationally intelligent." You will have an ever-evolving, failure-resistant HealthStyle that will change your life.

ELEVEN PROVEN STEPS TO MOTIVATION

STEP #1: *Not Fun, Not Done.* Enjoy the process; don't deprive yourself. Keep experimenting until you find foods and exercises that you sincerely like.

STEP #2: *Build Momentum.* Keep your program routine *consistent*, so your subconscious has time to "set" the new pattern. Give the new habits momentum by scheduling your workouts and planning your meals.

STEP #3: *Use Tools and Expertise.* Use progress charts, rewards, posted reminders and motivational signs, as well as the help of family, colleagues, and professionals for support. (See Habit Helpers, p. 95)

STEP #4: *Become an Expert on YOU.* Educate yourself about diet, exercise, and mental fitness. Tune in. Read. Keep updated.

STEP #5: *Plan Ahead.* Know that emergencies—daily, monthly and yearly—will arise. This should not be a continual surprise to you. Think ahead and develop alternatives for any situation.

STEP #6: *Evolutionary Approach.* Take it one step at a time and "upgrade" as you are ready. Be sure your program isn't complicated. Pace yourself and be patient. Set goals low enough to eliminate unnecessary pressure and ensure that you will always be a "success."

STEP #7: *Be Your Own Psychologist.* Analyze your resistance to exercise or dietary changes and learn to name and troubleshoot your obstacles. Use Self-Dialoguing to catch "errors in logic" and cultivate your own Trigger Statements (these are explained later).

STEP #8: *Take Control Without Guilt.* Prioritize, commit, develop discipline. Allow no excuses. But when you slip, err gracefully. Forgive yourself with a gentle, knowing smile and get right back on track.

STEP #9: *Tune in to your mind/body connection.* Use the scanning technique (also described later) for skill in feeling—physically and mentally—to experience your workouts, meals and life more fully.

STEP #10: *Reprogram Your Thoughts..* Learn to reprogram your mind to a positive point of view toward exercise and diet.

STEP #11: *Be Your Own Motivator.* Learn to be your own support system and best ally—not your own worst enemy.

Now let's examine the Eleven Proven Steps to Motivation more closely. Remember, these motivational building blocks are the foundation of your Healthy, Wealthy, & Wise Program and the keys to your success.

#1 Not Fun—Not Done

If not actually *fun*, exercise should at least be *satisfying*—at which point you have an excellent chance of getting it *done*. Take the time to find that special combination of time, place, and activities that makes exercise work for you, and your program can quite painlessly take care of itself. (Not surprisingly, studies show that participants in corporate programs have a better adherence record if they have a choice in fitness activities; in other words, if they tailor their workouts to their personal interests.) Think of exercise as a luxury, as an enrichment of your life, and seek out ways to make it more fulfilling, such as following up on the elites of your chosen sport, subscribing to magazines about it, taking lessons, getting a coach, or treating yourself to good equipment.

Regarding diet, while there are foods you definitely should avoid, you should think in terms of adding good foods rather than just taking away your coveted "no no's." The negatives will often tend to fade on their own as the positives take over. One executive told me of the time she decided to eliminate her last bad dietary habit—having a candy bar in the afternoon. She said it really wasn't that difficult, since she was pretty skilled at understanding the inner workings of motivation. "I made sure not to keep thinking 'Today consists of *not having a candy bar—all day!*' Instead, I went shopping for a special bowl, filled it with my favorite fruit, and put it on my desk. Now I grab a piece of fruit whenever I feel the candy bar urge. It works!"

Make every aspect of your HealthStyle fun and interesting. Think of it as a challenge to discover new hiking trails or tennis courts, health-oriented restaurants and grocery stores, versus the "splurge" mentality that says inactivity and eating fat-laden, refined foods is the ultimate reward.

Don't Deny Yourself.   Don't put yourself in mental and emotional jail. Making deep-rooted changes in your self-image and life goals is of the utmost importance because the self-denial approach doesn't work and is, in fact, destructive. For example, while you may deny yourself your favorite foods long enough to lose all the weight you want, those immortal foods are waiting in ambush to seduce you again as soon as you tire of your diet. That's why the failure rate is so high in the enrollment diet programs that abound. They are seductive in that they work—you *do* lose the weight, but 95 percent of the diets' participants also gain the weight back. Just remember this one inescapable truth: Self-denial makes up for itself *double*—like digging through the refrigerator with wild abandon at 3 A.M. In fact, a psychologist from the University of London found that the greatest abstainers were the greatest bingers—and the most overweight. Your good intentions haven't got a chance if you feel you are being punished. Not fun, not done.

#2 Build Momentum

Keep in mind that we reportedly forget 60 percent of any input within 24 hours (and up to 98 percent in one week). You can appreciate that we need constant input and regular reminders if we are to establish a HealthStyle pattern, especially in the beginning. One of the most common and most sincere excuses I hear with newcomers in my program at MCA/Universal is "I forgot." On the other hand, when your new HealthStyle approach becomes a habit, it will actually be disconcerting to alter it or skip it, just as it was initially difficult to pull away from the TV and the Twinkies.

The people I interviewed show that they believe in consistency. They keep exercise *frequency* high—five to seven days a week rather than three or four. Paul Oreffice of Dow Chemical is one exec who preaches what he practices: "To maintain a good program I believe consistency is important," he says. "Going on and off [your schedule] with vacations and weekends and so forth doesn't work." Train yourself as you would a child or even a dog—be consistent and give momentum a chance to build.

#3 Use Tools

Implement the tools in this book and any other resources that suit your needs: progress charts, rewards, music with exercise, spouse/ friend support, workout buddies, trainers, or coaches. Use Habit Helpers for support because, as I've mentioned, it's all too easy to "forget to remember" a new habit in the beginning stages of change. One client calls Habit Helpers her "alarm clocks." A few examples follow, but use your imagination and customize your own Habit Helpers to suit your particular circumstance.

HABIT HELPERS

1. Colored Dot Reminders.   When you are beginning to make (or break) a habit, place colored dot stickers (from a stationery store) in strategic locations: dashboard, refrigerator, bathroom mirror, kitchen sink, on the bottom of the TV frame, on your bedside table.

These repeated reminders will help you to internalize the habit. Remove them every two weeks, as you will stop noticing them (the habit will already have taken root by then). You can use different colors for different goals: purple for not snacking, neon yellow for thinking positively, and so forth. Tackle one habit at a time.

2. Motivational Phrases.   Write motivating reminders that apply to your particular goal on 5" × 7" cards (or larger) and post them in strategic locations:

On the refrigerator: "What you're looking for is not in here."

Next to your alarm clock: "Take **one** step" (a reminder to get up and at least take *one* tennis-shoed step out the door).

On your desk: "Relax" or "Breathe."

As you proceed in your program, you will quickly become adept at making up your own relevant, motivating phrases. If you prefer, you can put reminders in your own code so no one else knows what they mean. For example, a note on your dashboard could say "B Cool" and serve as a reminder to be like a calm Type B when rude drivers or slow traffic test your patience.

#4 Become an Expert on YOU

Educate yourself on diet and exercise basics, then keep yourself updated. This can be as simple as making sure to read related articles in your daily paper. Educating yourself about the positives and negatives of food and exercise will further motivate you to stick to your program, because you will understand the dynamics of your body—not just its capabilities but also its cravings and complaints. Be knowledgeable about *everything* that goes into your mouth. Choose salad dressing, sandwich spreads, and sauces carefully. Remember that frying foods doubles their calories and watch for calories in your beverages as well. If you *must* have that donut, fine, but perhaps it won't look as tasty if you are keenly aware that one plain donut (3.5 oz) has as many calories as four slices of bread with jam (about 400 calories), and 50 percent of the calories are from fat—versus only 10 percent fat calories for the bread and jam.

If you feel weak, hungry, or just plain miserable in the afternoon, it is useful if you understand that you may be feeling this way because your blood sugar has dropped. You will learn to realize that the remedy is not a jolt of caffeine or sugar (as they only temporarily boost blood sugar, which then drops lower than before) and you will be more likely to allow yourself a healthful snack, such as fruit or frozen nonfat yogurt, before you become ravenous and out of control.

In other words, being informed is key to self-motivation and part of your new HealthStyle effort—suffering is *not*.

#5 Plan Ahead

Always allow more time than you think you need and try to troubleshoot potential obstacles. (See Time Management Skills and How to Troubleshoot HealthStyle Obstacles in Chapter 6.)

#6 Take an Evolutionary Approach

Can't "cold turkey" the donuts? If you find it easier to climb Mount Everest than to cut out that breakfast donut, don't lose heart. You can keep your donut—for awhile. You may not be one of those people who can easily shift gears and head off in a new direction with food or anything else. Don't worry—even those who are flexible and highly motivated do better with a slow, modified approach. It's the tortoise-versus-the-hare theory. Just bite off what you can chew (so to speak) and gradually cut down. Specific evolutionary plans are outlined in the Diet and Exercise Programs.

1. Pace yourself.   Most of us know from experience by now that we can push something only so far—including ourselves. Why? Because we each have our own evolutionary pace within us that is, in fact, part of the greater force of nature. The important thing is to tune into that force, that pace, and flow with it instead of fighting it.

The successes I studied have, over the years, slowly refined and customized their individual HealthStyle efforts. They tackle one thing at a time—cutting down on red meat, for example. As new nutritional data becomes known, they revamp their programs accordingly and incorporate evolutionary thinking. Deciding that you "aren't allowed" to eat any junk food for the rest of your life can be depressing, especially on a bad day. Don't think about it. Just decide you are not going to indulge *today*. The farther away you get from something, the easier it becomes to let it go, provided you apply the relevant motivational tactics.

Here is a good pacing trick. Instead of always pushing yourself to the next level or getting caught up in making dramatic commitments, try holding yourself back before adding another element to your HealthStyle improvements. In other words, even after part of you is eager to add something (a half-mile run, for example) or quit something (sugar), wait another week or two to assure your readiness by building the anticipation, and commitment—and *plan*. For many, this creates a new, appreciative mindset that fuels motivation.

Recognize small victories (you skipped dessert three days in a row), but don't cling too hard to individual ups, downs, or plateaus.

Learn to ride the bumps for the long haul—or there will be no long haul. Instead of constantly pushing yourself, think "If this is all I *ever* do—it's okay, it's more than I was doing before." Remember, your diet and exercise program is not a contest with yourself or anyone else. At times, it may even be temporarily necessary to "evolve downward" to accommodate life's circumstances. See the whole picture objectively. I tell my clients to imagine their progress on a graph, with the jagged ups and downs, but with the overall movement being upward, as shown here.

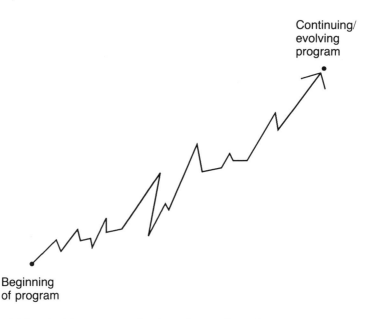

Continuing/
evolving
program

Beginning
of program

Take the Zen approach: Stay focused on the moment-to-moment process versus living for the results.

2. Set Modest Goals.   Set your goals one step lower than what you think you can do, because there is a difference between "can do" and "will do." Anything past that goal then becomes extra credit. Then, instead of thinking, "I really should be doing better," you can be thinking, "I'm really doing great. I'm a success." Goals that are too lofty can kill your efforts. In fact, to some people, goal-making of any kind represents pressure. Rather than set up "finish-line" goals such as, "I will lose ten pounds in thirty days," form a HealthStyle "plan" with clear-cut parameters, such as "I will walk three to four days a week for twenty to thirty minutes."

3. Be Patient.   There is an initial adjustment period for any new habit. It's like jumping into a swimming pool. At first, the water is cold, but it soon feels comfortable. Be patient. Give the new habit a chance to "catch" and have faith that it *will* become natural. You will soon "get in the habit of the habit." Patience is often the critical factor between success and failure.

4. Beware the All-or-Nothing Mentality.   Most people really don't understand the concept of moderation. That's understandable, since, from a very early age, we are fed an all-or-nothing mentality regarding practically everything, including exercise. We can spend $200 on the latest designer exercise attire, then run across town to our designer health club (which, when amortized, costs us about $25 per visit, since twenty visits is the average before quitting). We take an hour-long aerobics class and most likely leave with even lower self-esteem than when we arrived, having done jumping jacks behind some of the tightest derrieres in town. This drives us to struggle with the dreaded weight machines for another twenty to forty minutes so that we might look better for our next aerobics class (the same mentality that makes us clean the house before the maid comes). Finally, we take a sauna, get dressed and drive home, tired, sore, and frustrated. Our workout has consumed two to three hours of our precious time, and we have probably exercised too much, if anything. A twenty-minute walk suddenly seems worthless by comparison and is not even considered an option by avid health club aficionados. This is the all-or-nothing mentality that can sabotage even the most sincere intentions. Beware of it.

#7 Be Your Own Psychologist

To understand the mechanics of your thinking/behavior process, you must learn to figure out what goes askew in your inner control center (your subconscious)—and why. You must be able to hear your inner voice, the voice that says, "Oh, no, here we go again, another program that's going to take away my reason for living. I'll give it a week—max." That voice must be taken seriously. You must first *hear* it, then properly understand it, and then deal with it intelligently and sensitively. You can then better *analyze your resistance*. Why do you resist? Is it lack of commitment? Is a part of you determined to self-sabotage? (That is, you don't deserve to look and feel good, you have a fear of success, of achievement and recognition, of the opposite sex.) The resistance may be caused by a combination of these and other issues, but you don't necessarily need a therapist to find the answers. It is simply a matter of tuning in and being honest with yourself. You can learn to diagnose what triggers a slip in your motivation, name the specific roadblock (such as self-sabotage), and deal with it in an experienced and positive manner. You become an expert in troubleshooting your own problems. To eliminate continued failures, you must be able to recognize past programming, since that is the source of present problems.

HOW TO TROUBLESHOOT HEALTHSTYLE OBSTACLES

The following exercise can help you implement the number-one tactic for dealing with motivational slips: *identify the obstacle.* Once obstacles are exposed, they are much easier to eliminate. The chart below also can help you create your own strategy for eliminating obstacles altogether. The following is a typical Exercise Obstacle Chart. A few Motivational Solutions are filled in. For example, do only half of your workout when you are tired or sick. This is a solution to an exercise obstacle. Make your own diet and exercise obstacle lists. Then fill in the Motivational Solution column with solutions that best solve your particular obstacles. When the obstacles arise (and they will), you will have already solved them.

Sample: *Troubleshooting My Exercise Obstacles*

Obstacle	Motivational Solution
1. Tired, sick	1. I will do only half of my workout.
2. Bored	2. I'll add tennis to my weekend workout.
3. No time	3. (Fill in your own solutions.)
4. Depressed	4.
5. Inconvenient	5.
6. Bad weather	6.
7. Too fat (embarrassed)	7.

THREE SELF-DIALOGUING TECHNIQUES

Self-dialoguing enables you to contact your subconscious directly. Here are three useful techniques for employing self-dialoguing:

1. Use Trigger Statements.   Establish a repertoire of powerful words or phrases that will immediately and without fail remind you of the importance of your goals and bring you back to a motivational mentality in times of trouble. For example, when emotions make you want to binge, try countering with: "I won't let them (job, people, circumstances) make me fat." Or, "This (diet/exercise) is my choice."

2. Catch Errors in Logic.   A wise man once said, "Logic is the slave of passion." Unfortunately, we do allow our cravings (passions) or our aversions to play tricks with our ability to reason. An effective, self-dialoguing skill that helps you recognize and combat this phenomenon is to catch errors in your thinking process (logic) before acting on them. For example, consider this dialogue:

You #1: "It looks like rain. I better not walk today."
You #2: "Do you have an umbrella?"
You #1: "Yes, but . . ."
You #2: " 'But' nothing. Get the umbrella and let's go."
You #1: "Caught again. You win."

By continually exposing erroneous logic, your subconscious eventually will learn to no longer attempt such "logic."

You will learn to see the irony, the contradiction, of dodging your own HealthStyle. It is a matter of deciding that you *want* to change these habits, not just *need* to. It is your *choice*. Think of your efforts to improve your HealthStyle as nurturing a luxury you deserve—health and success—and not as a self-imposed bootcamp. This rings true to the now-popular concept of "being your own parent," currently touted by psychologists and self-help programs. In this approach, you essentially assume the role of a devoted parent whose main concern is taking care of *you*.

3. Apply Exer-Psychology. This is the term I use to describe self-dialoguing when acting as your own exercise analyst. It actually encompasses the above two techniques, but covers motivational aspects, as well. The fact is, when (not "if") the physical pain, discomfort, inconvenience, or boredom induced by exercise becomes too much, the mind will rebel. The subconscious will simply take over and find reasons to "ease" exercise back out of your life. Using exer-psychology can alleviate this response.

One of the main exercise dilemmas, especially for beginners, is that of knowing when to give yourself permission to alter your program. There is a fine line between pushing too hard and not pushing hard enough. When do you "listen to your body" and heed its message, as in "Skip it—you've had a hard day and life is rough . . ."? Or when do you say to yourself, "Yes, it's tough, yes, I'm tired—but I'm committed to this workout . . ."? The answer is actually pretty basic and again has to do with habits. It is this: Don't trust yourself until you have 60 to 90 days of good program in your HealthStyle bank account. Once again, give the momentum a chance to build. Until that time, don't listen to any excuse except your doctor's. (And if you must cut back, remember that reducing exercise duration and intensity is more acceptable than reducing frequency.) The mind is very sneaky and will try to con you back to your old comfort zone, especially on tired or busy days. Use exer-psychology. Tell yourself, "This is where most people fall off, but *I'm* not most people." Except for dire conditions, you must not listen until you are hooked (routinized) on your program. Put your mind on hold and put your body into action.

Malcolm Stamper of Boeing says he loves the challenge of pushing himself. He has figured out the whole exer-psychology approach on his own. The point, he says, is that people give the wrong reasons for not exercising, such as boredom. Boredom, he says, is the wrong description—"The mind is saying 'I don't want to do this,' and you translate that semantically into boredom." Malcolm agrees that the mind can be a powerful tool working against you and adds, "The way to get around it is strictly a mental trick. Say to yourself 'Hang in there a little longer and get past the unpleasant point to the high.' Your body will throw out a few endorphins, and you'll think you've had a martini. Then you'll say, 'Gee, I'd like to get to that point again.' "

The hazy line between pushing too hard and not pushing hard enough becomes clearer as your HealthStyle improvement efforts become a habit. As you gain true intimacy with your body, you will become more adept at knowing when to pull back and when to push.

#8 Take Control Without Guilt

Four Ways to Take Control.   You (and only you) are responsible for yourself and any changes that are going to take place in your life. Take control and make them happen. The following four methods can help:

1. *Prioritize.* Your program must come first—*you* must come first. This is a strange new concept for many people.

2. *Commit.* Decide that health *works* and is a consequential investment of time and energy. Until the momentum of the program kicks in to help motivate you, make your program priorities simple and clear. Write them down and tell your friends, but, most important, keep telling yourself. Commit to a little extra time at first to give the program a chance to "catch." It will soon take off on its own. If possible, begin at a time that will allow you 60 to 90 days of relative low tension and minimal travel, so you can focus on your new HealthStyle goals.

3. *Be Disciplined.* Regardless of how interesting or fun you make your HealthStyle improvement efforts, at times you

may still need some old-fashioned discipline, especially in the beginning. If you weren't taught discipline as a child, you must find it, develop it, and nurture it. If your efforts are right for you and you are properly armored psychologically, however, discipline will become second nature and habit will soon take over. In the beginning, though, grab hold of your new habit like a bulldog. Stay with it. Don't allow lapses. Don't "forget" how important this is to you. Discipline helps you keep your priorities clear.

4. *Don't Make Excuses.* Excuses are the most common downfall with any new program and are a definite threat to the most sincere "priority list." Excuses must be mercilessly confronted. It's not always fun to confront excuses, but confronting them *does* get easier with practice. My father used to confront our excuses for us. When trying to squirm our way out of his piano practice or homework interrogation (with what I thought were praiseworthy excuses), he would interrupt with, "What's the bottom line—did you do it or didn't you?" I will never forget those moments of truth that wouldn't go away. The practice or the homework either was done or it wasn't. Period. And the consequences were not pleasant—such as having to stay home from the school dance. I learned at an early age that your actions show up in black and white and that no excuse can transform black into white.

Recently, as I was "exploring" a client's excuses with her, I watched her frustration build. When she finally reached the "dead end of excuses," she turned to me and burst out, "I hate you—you make me face myself!" Uncomfortable as this was, she had come face to face with her self-defeating excuse-making. Perhaps for the first time she realized she had to assume complete responsibility for every aspect of her life, to take control. She needn't try to outsmart a calorie chart, the scale, me—or herself. Many people spend a lifetime avoiding this frightening but ultimately freeing realization, but it is the key to honest, healthy living. The next time you feel you *HAVE* to eat a piece of fudge, made by the resident office goodie-maker, "to spare her feelings," ask yourself who you're trying to kid. Remember that your bathroom scale has a "bottom line" and that it doesn't hear excuses very well.

Dealing with Guilt.   While you must take control and be firm with yourself at times, it is also important to eliminate the word *guilt* from your vocabulary. Learn to err gracefully. Once in awhile, you'll have a bad day and will just have to accept it. Understand this as an exception to the rule (versus another uncontrollable downward spiral). You must learn to break the habit of waking up feeling like a degenerate felon because you ate too much of Aunt Myrtle's divinity fudge last night. For one thing, life is too short to inflict yourself with bad feelings. For another, guilt breeds more binges. So catch that moment of mental flogging and replace it with positive internal feedback, such as "Even though I overate yesterday, I'm still a good person, and I don't need to punish myself with starvation or bingeing today." If you are guilt-prone, make a sign for your mirror that says *No Guilt Allowed.*

#9 Tune In to Your Mind-Body Connection

Our habits and personality traits limit us and are products of past experiences. The Sanskrit word for this history is *samskaras.* Very simply, samskaras are the psychological knots that are formed throughout our lives. They are our conditioning, and they manifest themselves in the form of cravings and aversions. Every aspect of your life is ruled to some degree by these cravings and aversions, and together they create one's personality and habits. "Scanning" is a style of an age-old meditation technique called vipassana that helps you dissolve the knots of your past. Scanning means just that—a systematic scan (or close examination) of your body. You can mentally scan your entire body from head to toe or select a certain area to scan. Scanning teaches you to experience your body in a new way; it redefines "getting in touch with yourself" and can thereby short-circuit the usual program relapses.

Scanning can teach you to experience life 100 percent—minute by minute. Unfortunately, most people spend their lives never fully conscious. One third of your life is spent completely unconscious—sleeping. The other two thirds is spent in a surface level of consciousness, dealing with day-to-day business. Scanning helps you be mindful, to be fully aware, and to *experience* life completely. Vipassana teacher Shinzen Young believes that by constantly expanding your consciousness and awareness, the inner growth rate of an adult can be equal to that of a child. In this sense, you become a "super adult" instead of simply an old child with gray hair.

1. Scanning and Exercise.   Exercise with awareness and experience your body in a whole new way. Scan (observe) your body one part at a time, from head to toe or just the most prominent area of the moment (feet when running, arms when lifting weights). Be aware of your breath as you scan. Feel the rhythm of air entering and exiting your body for your entire workout. You might finish with a free-form scan of the whole body. Fully feel every movement and sensation (accomplished athletes often tune in to the *experience* of the exercise rather than using distractions, such as exercise buddies or music).

2. Scanning and Diet.   Eat with awareness. Too often, we eat while distracted, and thus we do not fully enjoy the process. We tend to engage in a mindless sort of stuffing process, not because our bodies are still hungry, but because our minds haven't been satisfied and are detached from our bodies. Our mind says, "keep it coming," because it wasn't completely conscious when the first load went down, so we eat more, distracted and half aware. And so the cycle goes— and the bathroom scale creeps up.

Instead, combat the urge to eat fast. Eat alone in quiet as often as possible, especially for the first few weeks, and work on integrating mouth and stomach—eating and consciousness. Try to be aware of each bite, savoring the feel in your mouth, the full flavor of it, the pleasurable sensations spreading to the whole body. And learn to detect the slightest hint of feeling satisfied (versus full). Stop eating at that point. Then feel the afterglow of tastes throughout the body, or perhaps a certain sadness that all the good tastes and fun are over. Take a moment to locate and scan the physical sensations of this sadness in your body (throat, chest, stomach, and so forth). Feel the sadness completely, and it will dissipate. Also, remind yourself that you get to eat again in just a few hours—this is not your last meal on earth.

Scanning develops eating, exercising, and living with *awareness*. With practice, you will eat less and enjoy it more; exercise more and enjoy it more—and live life more completely. Scanning is further described in Chapter 7, Mental Fitness Training.

#10 Reprogram Your Thoughts

Most programs fail (notice I said *programs* fail, not *you* fail) because they don't alter your "core problem," whether it's a distaste for exercise or a fatal attraction to a particular food. One technique that effectively makes deep-rooted changes without self-denial is re-programming your thoughts, or "brainwashing." Brainwashing is a light little term I use to describe a very important motivational technique: using images or facts to reverse your thinking in a certain area. With it you can literally and permanently make a good thing appear bad and vice versa.

Mind Over Mouth is brainwashing as applied to diet. Mind Over Mouth enables you to permanently change your taste buds and comfortably eliminate dietary villains. One business owner said she actually "brainwashed" herself into detesting the smell and taste of her former addiction, fried chicken. This technique is something you can do yourself quite easily. Pick any food that has you hooked and do some creative imagery. With greasy fast food, you can imagine the rancid, carcinogenic oil they use (over and over again) coagulating its way through your blood stream. Look at the food and think of it in negative terms, even if you don't believe such images will work. Imagine the greasy stomachache it gives you (as if you've just drunk a cup of the frying oil straight). If that image isn't strong enough, you might want to shoot straight to a scene where you are getting bypass surgery for those clogged arteries. Every time you see or smell the food, go to work on your imagery. With the proper concentration, consistency, and diligence, you should notice a difference by ten imagery sessions.

This technique is effective because the subconscious doesn't really know the difference between visualization and actualization (reality). It will believe anything you tell it. You'll find brainwashing much easier than trying to hold your breath around tempting foods for a lifetime. Be sure to apply brainwashing in reverse, as well. Make healthful things more appealing, such as foods for which you want to acquire a taste (fresh, crispy salads and the delicate taste of uncooked greenery unpolluted by fatty salad dressings), or exercise (imagine how good it makes you look and feel).

#11 Be Your Own Motivator

Acknowledge your achievements. *Be Positive.* This principle is basic but also very much underused. In fact, it is said that 80 percent of our internal dialogue is negative. This much negative input produces negative emotional states that, not coincidentally, are a major cause of relapses. Learn how to pump yourself up when setbacks occur or when you just can't seem to get going (see motivation step #7, Self-Dialoguing). At the age of 74, my father, an avid golfer, decided that he wanted to hit across the lake on the seventeenth hole (he says, "The old ones can't hit over the lake from the tee"). Without telling anyone his plan, he started doing pushups to build strength in his upper body. He worked up to one hundred pushups a day (fifty at a time)—the last ten being nearly impossible. He later told me that thinking of the lake would get him through the last ten pushups each day. What might be boring calisthenics to someone else became a personal Olympics for Dad. And yes, there's a great finish to the story. After six months, Dad hit his first ball over the lake!

Be your own motivator, your own support system, and your best ally, not your worst enemy.

Part Two

TAKING ACTION:

THE HWW HEALTHSTYLE PROGRAM

My wife and I are healthier in our sixties than we were in our forties. It's a way of life that we truly love.

—*Malcolm Stamper, Boeing*

INTRODUCTION TO PART II

STRATEGIES FOR ACHIEVING HEALTH— AND SUCCESS

> The "key" to a healthy life is BALANCE. Balance is how we work, how we play, what we eat, when we eat, and, most importantly, a balanced, healthy attitude about those around us and about ourselves.
> —William Howell, CEO, CB, J. C. Penney

Two Steps to a Better HealthStyle

You are most likely reading this book because you've already made the decision to upgrade your current quality of life. And by now you should be convinced that these execs are doing something that pays off in a big way. Being convinced is Step 1. Step 2 is doing it.

The good news, as you have seen, is that "doing it" is relatively easy. The successes I studied take a practical, common-sense approach to fitness. In two key words, they are *consistent*, and they use *moderation*. This makes it easy for you, because consistency and moderation do not demand superhuman willpower or turning your life upside down. Remember, at the start of *any* program, ask yourself, "Can I live with this indefinitely?" The beauty of the HWW HealthStyle Program is that it is not only one you *can* do, but it is one you *will* do—and keep doing, because it is adaptable, enjoyable, and effective. It *works—you just need to commit, make it fun, and hang in there.*

THE FOUR ELEMENTS OF THE HWW HEALTHSTYLE PROGRAM

The HWW HealthStyle Program is divided into four parts:

1. Motivation Timeline
2. Mental Fitness (Stress Management) Program
3. Diet Program
4. Exercise Program

I find it most effective to use all four programs interactively, but they also work well alone. Don't think you have to do all four or none at all. For example, if you want to start with diet and think about exercise later, fine. Do what will work best for you. I would, however, like to suggest a few particularly complementary program combinations. For example, exercise is especially helpful when dieting. Studies at Baylor Institute showed that participants kept weight off when exercise was included with dieting. When participants only dieted the weight returned within two years.

Primary Program (Your Main Focus)	Especially Complementary Program(s) (Helps Your Progress)
Stress Management Program	Exercise Program
Diet Program	Motivation, Stress Management and Exercise Program
Exercise Program	Motivation Program

SAMPLE *HWW* HEALTHSTYLE PROGRAMS

Here are the programs of two top executives in my study. Their commitment and consistency will help to inspire you to take action.

DAVID MILLER
President, Emeritus
J. C. Penney

Vital Stats:

Weight: 160

Height: 5'9½

Chol: 160

BP: 140/88

Vitamins: C, A, D, codliver oil

Coffee: None

Cigarettes: No

Alcohol: Has one drink per day.

Stress/Attitude: Handles stress by "getting away." Thinks positively by "talking myself into things."

David's Typical Daily Diet

Meal	Time	Food	Calories per Meal
Breakfast	7	yogurt	
		blueberries	
		or cabbage and carrots	
		or oatmeal	350
Lunch	12	grilled snapper	
		green salad	
		bran muffin	400
Snack	5	½ banana	45
Dinner	8	chicken	
		carrots	
		rice	
		wine (one glass)	650
		TOTAL	1445

COMMENTS:

David eats no sugar. Notice how low David's cholesterol is. Now notice the cholesterol-lowering foods he eats: carrots, oatmeal, rice, fish. David says his weight has never been a problem, and you can see why from his diet.

David's Weekly Exercise

Activity	Duration	Frequency	Calories Used
swimming	30 min.	5× week	210 × 5 = 1050
stretching	10 min.	3× week	35 × 3 = 105
chin-ups	5 min.	3× week	35 × 3 = 105
golf	90 min.	1× week	270
			WEEKLY TOTAL = 1530

"ROCKY" JOHNSON
CEO, Chairman of the Board
GTE

Vital Stats:

Weight: 177
Height: 5'9½
Chol: 275
BP: 134/76
Vitamins: None
Coffee: Drinks decaf
Cigarettes: Smokes an occasional cigar
Alcohol: Has about four drinks per week.

COMMENTS:

Exercise is Rocky's sleeping pill. "Exercise relieves me of stress at the end of the day and it clears up my mind," he says. "It also helps me sleep a lot better."

Rocky's secretary says "He puts me to shame [healthwise], and I'm twenty years younger!" Rocky had a health scare with hypertension sixteen years ago, which he manages through exercise, and he also continually watches his cholesterol. Rocky's parents taught him the hard-work ethic, and he believes "aspiring is good for you." Duck carving is his creative hobby. He also enjoys playing bridge.

Rocky's Typical Daily Diet

Meal	Time	Food	Calories per Meal
Breakfast	7	cereal	
		fruit	
		decaf	295
Lunch	11	soup	
		salad	350
Snack	6	cheese and crackers	250
Dinner	7:30	fish	
		vegetable	
		potato	375
Snack	9	pineapple	60
		TOTAL	1330

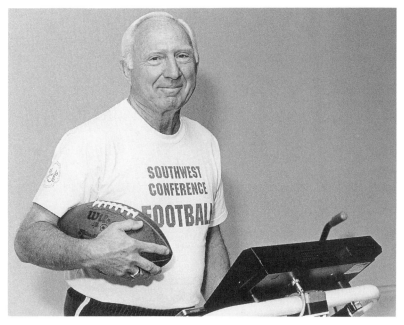

J.L. "Rocky" Johnson, CEO and Chairman of the Board of GTE, maintains a rigorous fitness schedule that warrants his nickname.

Rocky's Weekly Exercise

Activity	Duration	Frequency	Calories Used
Jogging	40 min.	2× week (on weekends)	240 × 2 = 480
Nautilus	20 min.	5× week	140 × 5 = 700
Treadmill	30 min.	5× week	180 × 5 = 900
Stretch	5 min.	7× week	20 × 7 = 140
Tennis	60 min.	1× week	360
Golf	90 min.	1× week	270
			WEEKLY TOTAL = 2850

(Occasionally replaces jogging/treadmill with rowing machine or exercycle.)

DON'T RACE— PACE

MANAGING YOUR TIME FOR HEALTH AND SUCCESS

My lists have lists.

—*Columbe Nicholas, Christian Dior*

FOUR CRUCIAL TIME MANAGEMENT RULES

Before launching into your efforts to improve your Health-Style, you may need some basic skills in time management. Without them, even the best program hasn't got a chance. Give the following time management strategy some consideration before beginning your HealthStyle improvement efforts.

People who most need time management guidance are usually too busy or too disorganized to read entire books on the subject. It's just as well. Some of the complex systems of time management I have seen could turn an innocent, relaxed Type B into a full-fledged, eye-twitching Type A, if it were possible. While effective for many, elaborate time management systems can take others an abundance of time just planning their time.

The truth is that time management is fairly basic. The first rule is that you must start being brutally *honest* with yourself. You need to stop overscheduling yourself or overestimating what you can accomplish in a set period of time. Be realistic about the number of minutes in an hour and the number of hours in a day. And don't play games, such as setting your watch ahead. If you are habitually late, vow that from now on, your goals for what you will accomplish in a given day will be one notch lower (more realistic) than what your former self would set and that you will keep this "contract" with yourself. The next time you catch yourself starting to cram in one more thing when you should be leaving, stop in your tracks, get up and leave on time—*no matter what*. You will learn to ignore the erroneous logic of your "late self." You will simply walk out that door, with no argument. If you do this consistently, you will eventually break the late habit.

The second rule is that you must *prioritize* the things that fill your life. For example, many of the leaders in this book emphasize that they schedule their workout on their daily calendar, just as they would a business appointment. Their secretaries are instructed to schedule appointments around this time, if at all possible. Similarly, the participants with the best results in my program at MCA/Universal continually impress me with the importance they give their HealthStyle program. Since it takes place during their lunch break (three days a week), there are many tempting as well as demanding appointments that must be rescheduled to accommodate it. "This program has become a way of life for me," said one.

Randy Barron has many priorities and has learned that he can balance them quite effectively when he sticks to his plan. He runs a major corporation (Southwestern Bell), spends time with his family, and exercises regularly. One sacrifice is TV. Randy says, "I don't let the TV get to me at night—too many fall into that trap." Start improving your time management skills by making a list of priorities and include everything from exercise to business to family.

The third rule is that you must conquer *procrastination*. The tendency to procrastinate is particularly common when goals are unclear or seem overwhelming. The Personal Goals Chart can help you define attainable goals. However, the main thing procrastinators need to remember is to somehow *start* the thing *now*. Make a sign for your desk (taped to the front of a picture frame) that says Begin Now. I have found this simple tool amazingly effective. Once the job is started, the battle is half over.

I once worked with a successful attorney who had allowed himself to fall three years behind on his taxes. While he dealt with the problems of his clients competently, he had relinquished control over much of his personal life. As we worked on exercise and diet, I could see him building the "strength" to face his taxes. In 20 days he had lost 8½ pounds and was breaking a sweat for 30 to 45 minutes, five days a week.

I finally asked him if he felt ready to tackle his tax task. He said "Yes," but I wasn't convinced. I didn't ask him about it again for two weeks. When I did, he had not yet started. This little dance went on for another month and a half before I suggested that he *begin now*, with me there for moral support. I actually sat in his office with him on a Saturday so there would be no interruptions, and we painstakingly began. (The phone rang about six times but I didn't allow him to answer it.) I am anything but a tax expert, but I know what getting bogged down looks like and I know what *expedite* means. I kept him moving for four hours until we had one year of taxes accountant-ready. He couldn't believe that after all this time he had made so much progress in so little time. And, thus motivated, he finished the rest on his own within the week. He now pulls out his Begin Now sign whenever he feels the slightest hint of procrastination about anything.

The fourth, and perhaps the most important, rule is to *ENJOY THE PROCESS*. It's sometimes easier to assess what you can and cannot do if you promise yourself that you can do everything—one thing at a time—*if* and *when* time permits. Once you see how smoothly your life runs, you will think twice about the old "cram it all in" method of time management. After all, if you're always rushing around and running late, you can't be enjoying the process of living, so it doesn't really matter how much you fit in a day, does it?

Redken's CEO, Paula Kent Meehan, used to have trouble holding herself back from too many activities. "I really, sincerely, deeply believe I can do anything. And I've been a lot of things, like a contractor, and things that of course I had no business doing, but I *had* to do them. One day, a friend said to me 'Maybe you can do *any*thing, but you can't do *every*thing.' So every now and then, I stop myself and say 'Maybe I'm able to do this, but I can't do it if I'm doing these other things, too.' " *Remember to enjoy the process of living.*

HOW TO MAKE TIME VISUAL USING "TIMELINES"

If you have trouble with the concept of time, the following timeline will help you. Total your hours for each activity in a typical week and then take inventory. This is quick, visual, and very rewarding. In other words, add up the hours already accounted for in your day and week and see what is "left over" for other things. This will enable you to spot where you can cut down on the time wasters and where you can be more productive with your time. Once you've established an unbiased and realistic picture of your timeline on paper, you will most likely realize that you are not focusing enough attention on any one area and are consistently having limited success in *all* areas. Don't skip over this exercise—it is a quick and effective tool and one that is easy to implement. Incidentally, I find most people are commonly overextended anywhere from a half to one and a half days.

Here's what you do:

1. First, assign a time estimate to each activity (see Weekly Timeline Guide).

2. Then, go through each day of the week and assign the *actual time spent* doing each activity (Daily Timeline). Be honest and extra generous with your "actual time" entries. Keep records for a week on "Daily Timeline Guide." Remember, tasks such as picking up dry cleaning include travel time and waiting time.

3. Add up the subtotals of all seven days. Enter them in your Weekly Timeline "Reality" column. Now compare that weekly total with your original estimate. (For biweekly or monthly items, treat your time entries as if this were the week for them.)

4. Finally, set your New Goal (Weekly Timeline) after you've assessed "the evidence."

Weekly Timeline Guide

	Estimate	Reality	New Goal
Total Hours in a Week:	168	168	168
Subtract:			
Sleep (Sample 7 × 7 hours/night = 49)	49	45.5	52.5
Personal care (dress, shower, shave, facial, hairdresser, nails)	_____	_____	_____
Exercise (dress, shower, drive time)	_____	_____	_____
Eat (preparation, drive, wait time, etc.)	_____	_____	_____
Work (drive time, overtime, etc.)	_____	_____	_____
Duties (pay bills, errands, shop, etc.)	_____	_____	_____
Housecleaning	_____	_____	_____
Laundry	_____	_____	_____
Grocery shopping	_____	_____	_____
Family time (include time alone with spouse)	_____	_____	_____
Entertainment (friends, movies, fun, etc.)	_____	_____	_____
Hobbies, study, classes, etc.	_____	_____	_____
Sports	_____	_____	_____
"Veg" time (do nothing, read, TV, etc.)	_____	_____	_____
Relaxation (meditation, massage, etc.)	_____	_____	_____
Other: (appointments—dentist, doctor, charity, school, etc.)	_____	_____	_____
	_____	_____	_____
	_____	_____	_____
	_____	_____	_____
Total hours left after subtracting above	_____	_____	_____

Daily Timeline Guide

(Photocopy and complete for each day of the week)

Day _____

	Reality	New Goal
Hours in Day:	24	24
Subtract:		
Sleep	_____	_____
Personal care (dress, shower, shave, facial, hairdresser, nails)	_____	_____
Exercise (dress, shower, drive time)	_____	_____
Eat (preparation, drive, wait time, etc.)	_____	_____
Work (drive time, overtime, etc.)	_____	_____
Duties (pay bills, errands, shop, etc.)	_____	_____
Housecleaning	_____	_____
Laundry	_____	_____
Grocery shopping	_____	_____
Family time (include time alone with spouse)	_____	_____
Entertainment (friends, movies, fun, etc.)	_____	_____
Hobbies, study, classes, etc.	_____	_____
Sports	_____	_____
"Veg" time (do nothing, read, TV, etc.)	_____	_____
Relaxation (meditation, massage, etc.)	_____	_____
Other:	_____	_____
	_____	_____
	_____	_____
	_____	_____
Total hours left after subtracting above	_____	_____

Travel Checklist

TOILETRIES

Shaving equipment ⎯⎯⎯

Glasses, contact lens spares and cleaning supplies ⎯⎯⎯

Makeup ⎯⎯⎯

Toothbrush/paste ⎯⎯⎯

Hair: brush, spray, dryer, shampoo, gel, curlers, etc. ⎯⎯⎯

CLOTHES

Shirts, blouses ⎯⎯⎯

Pants, skirts ⎯⎯⎯

Ties, belts, accessories ⎯⎯⎯

Shoes, socks, hosiery ⎯⎯⎯

Underwear ⎯⎯⎯

Evening wear ⎯⎯⎯

Coat, hat, gloves, scarf ⎯⎯⎯

Exercise gear ⎯⎯⎯

Misc: swimsuit, etc. ⎯⎯⎯

OTHER

Business supplies: phone numbers, files ⎯⎯⎯

Vitamins, prescription drugs ⎯⎯⎯

Snacks (nutritious) ⎯⎯⎯

Miscellaneous: ⎯⎯⎯

⎯⎯⎯

⎯⎯⎯

⎯⎯⎯

⎯⎯⎯

⎯⎯⎯

⎯⎯⎯

A TIMESAVING TRAVEL CHECKLIST

Since staying on a program while traveling is a challenge to almost everybody, I have included a simple but effective Travel Checklist that will help you save time, keep organized, and stay sane. Feel fee to add items of your own and photocopy for regular use.

TIPS TO REMEMBER:

- *Be brutally honest with yourself about time.*
- *Prioritize the things that fill your life.*
- *Conquer procrastination—Begin now!*
- *Enjoy the process versus "cram it all in."*

BE
YOUR OWN
MOTIVATOR

Chapter Seven

A BETTER HEALTHSTYLE STARTS IN YOUR HEAD

MENTAL FITNESS TRAINING

Keep everything in balance. If you neglect a part of your life—your personal life or your family—it causes mental stress.
—*Rocky Johnson, CEO, CB, GTE*

This chapter shows how the leaders in this book deal with stress. I also define the various types of stress and provide some tips for dealing with them. After you have been "stress educated," you will be ready for the Mental Fitness Program that follows.

WHY YOU NEED A POSITIVE MINDSET

According to a Harvard University report, ignoring stress will kill you just as easily as ignoring your dietary or exercise requirements. In fact, the *American Journal of Health Promotion* has reported that *60 to 90 percent of all medical visits are linked to stress.* Among other things, current research indicates a connection between high levels of stress and elevated cholesterol and blood pressure levels,

127

along with weakened immune systems. A suppressed immune system means that your body forms more free radicals. Increased free radical formation means a faster aging process. The bottom line: *stress accelerates the aging process.*

Studies show that Americans are doing more to prevent accidents and disease but are actually doing less to reduce stress. Stress management has not yet been given the same "press" as seat belts or air bags, for example, although stress can be just as debilitating as many major preventable accidents or diseases.

In my study I found that a positive mindset has helped America's highest-ranked view stress with a perspective that is radically different from the average American's. In fact, an impressive 78 percent of these men and women either work on positive thinking or claim it comes to them naturally. Those who follow established techniques turn to meditation, Norman Vincent Peale, Dale Carnegie and the Bible, among other sources of inspiration.

Some of the successes in my study claim to be natural positive thinkers, while others admit that they have to work at staying positive. Positive thinking comes naturally to Eileen Ford, head of the top modeling agency that bears her name. "I don't brood—I never look back," she says. In some respects these men and women are simply reflecting the confidence that comes with being at the top. But the ability to handle pressure gracefully is undoubtedly one of the reasons they have come so far.

Many also credit their upbringing for their positive attitude. For example, Redken's CEO, Paula Kent Meehan, says, "My mother is the most positive person in the world. Every meal she eats is the *best* meal she's ever had. I believe in being positive and creative about opportunities. in other words, if something can't be done one way, instead of getting frustrated, I think of a way it *can* be done."

Coca-Cola's Brian Dyson says his favorite maxim for dealing with stress is "don't sweat the small stuff." He adds, with a smile, "It's mostly small stuff." Charles Kittrell favors a *can-do* maxim: "If you want your prayers answered, get up off your knees and hustle."

There's another perspective to the "be positive" story that I think is worth mentioning. Positivism can be taken to unrealistic, out-of-touch extremes by people who can't deal with negativity and are in denial. It's important for your mental health to admit when things aren't going well and not feel guilty for being human.

HOW THE SUCCESSFUL TAKE BETTER CARE OF THEIR MINDS

While you may well be above the American norm in your

ability to handle stress and stay mentally fit, it is still shocking (and, hopefully, motivating) to contrast the men and women I interviewed with the average American. According to one study, only 20 percent of Americans say they enjoy life and are happy. In fact, one out of every four people will require some kind of psychological therapy before age 40. Stress is one of the biggest causes of psychological problems for Americans. Stress-related illnesses cost U.S. businesses at least 500 million employee workdays a year.

In contrast, 88 percent of those I studied say they handle stress well. On their way to the top, they decided that stress management deserved priority, and the majority say that they have gotten better at dealing with stress. Most are now able to recognize when they are under stress, and have developed specific ways to handle it.

Armco's CEO emeritus, Bob Boni, says: "You can handle a great deal of stress if you are in charge of your life. That's one of the joys of being CEO." But what do they do when they don't have control? Sam Schwartz of Conoco is "okay with stress because I don't worry about things over which I have no control." But most people *do* worry. According to Cornell University Medical College, those who feel little control over their jobs are three times as likely to develop hypertension. The participants in my study started at the bottom just as the rest of us did. One important reason that they have made it to the top is that they have learned how to deal with the demands placed upon them.

Type B's.   Contrary to the findings of "upper-level management" studies, corporate heads in my study are Type B's (confident, friendly, relaxed). In fact, a surprisingly low 5 percent of the men have Type A behavior (long associated with high-power executives), compared to an astounding 75 percent of urban American males who fit into the Type A category. The fact that these busy men and women took valuable time from their workdays for my interviews and follow-up conversations attests to their open, Type B natures. Their relaxed openness also shows that the hard, cold, "time is money" mentality traditionally associated with America's corporate giants is definitely *not* the credo of these leaders.

Opinions vary on defining Type A, as many now feel that we are all a combination of Types and categorization is not so simple. But while there are varieties and nuances within and between the types, it usually boils down to being more one than another—either relaxed and slower paced (Type B) or higher strung and faster paced (Type A). Being a recovering Type A myself, however, I am going to stick with the original Type A definition, while I agree there are degrees involved. Type A's are, to one degree or another, aggressive, uptight, and often harbor feelings of hostility. These traits, especially hostility, are thought to raise blood levels of triglyceride, cholesterol, ACTH, and norepinephrine. (In case these terms remind you of a nightmare college course, they simply mean that being a Type A can be bad for your health.)

Better Marriages.   Being Type B's could help explain why these HWW leaders are better mates, as well. Type A behavior raises divorce rates, with 50 percent of Type A marriages ending in divorce, compared with a 2 percent divorce rate for the men and women in this book. In fact, the executives in this study have been married an impressive 22½ years longer, on average, than the rest of us! This is a relevant health factor, since statistics show that married men and women aged 45 to 64 are healthier than their peers who are divorced, separated, widowed, or have never married. This may be because the immune systems of married people function better, according to one study. Charles Kittrel of Phillips Petroleum says, "I handle stress well today, but I had to learn how over the years." One way he relaxes is by taking long walks with his wife of 40 years. (Statistics also show that couples who exercise together stay with HealthStyle improvement programs longer.)

HOW TO KEEP A POSITIVE MINDSET: THE TIN MAN THEORY

"Think you can, think you can't—either way you'll be right."
—Anonymous

Starting to feel inadequate? No need. The purpose of this book is not to tell you how the other half lives and leave you paralyzed with the discrepancy. The message is that you can also achieve all that you were meant to—without a lobotomy, starvation, or monastic living—and actually enjoy the process. Remember the Scarecrow, the Cowardly Lion and the Tin Man in *The Wizard of Oz,* who wanted respectively a brain, courage and a heart? It took them a long yellow brick road and a harrowing soul-searching journey (not to mention two hours of TV time) to discover they possessed these qualities all along. The same goes for you. You have the resources—they just need to be tapped. But if you don't believe you possess the innate resources to get fit or achieve success, you probably won't. Allan Belzer, president, Allied Signal, says, "Self-image and staying fit is a circular situation. If you aren't fit, you can lean toward low self-esteem and if you have low self-esteem you are less apt to exercise and stay fit." Conversely, just the *idea* of taking care of your body is said to boost self-esteem, which gives you the confidence to try harder in other areas (career).

TIPS FROM THE TOP: HOW YOU (& YOUR DOG) CAN BEAT STRESS

Do America's highest-ranked ever feel stressed? Of course. "You go through times when you're on your brink of total capacity every day," says Kay Koplovitz. "That's when you can blow out, and then you can have medical problems." Sticking your neck out and working at your peak on a continual basis will get you ahead, no doubt about it, but it can also take its toll on your health if you're not careful. This is especially true as you get older. As Marcia Israel, founder of Judy's, puts it: "As you get older, your shock absorbers get a little thinner." We all have varying reactions to stress and different levels of tolerance to stress. The point is that everybody is subjected to stress these days. (The other day I even saw a dog scampering straight down the middle of the sidewalk, head and tail down, "all business," as if he was late for an appointment. The only thing missing was a briefcase.)

In sharp contrast to most of the American public, the majority of the HWW leaders have found ways to vent frustration and manage stress when it comes up. As you remember, most of the men in this book say that exercise works best for releasing stress. "The terror of going down ski slopes makes me forget about my troubles," says Brian Dyson of Coca-Cola. Mental health professionals concur; they are increasingly recommending exercise programs instead of drugs for their patients who are hypertensive or depressed.

Many of the women in my study use exercise as a release for stress, as well. Gilda Marx says, "My walks are more of a mental exercise—the physical just happens to go along for the walk." "I'm a Type A," admits Kay Koplovitz. "I'm aggressive and I can't stand being behind a car in traffic." Kay takes care of tension buildup by heading straight for the gym after work. "I release all that tension and get rid of it, then I feel better."

But the women also have other methods for coping with stress. "I like to cook when I'm under stress," says Columbe Nicholas, president emeritus of Christian Dior. "I chop and dice and use the Cuisinart—I do something menial with my hands." Like most of the others, however, Columbe doesn't put added pressure on herself. She has no room for guilt when she doesn't have time to prepare a meal. "I'm the first one to say: 'Okay, let's order Chinese.' " Besides exercise, Gilda Marx admits, "I also like to do something silly, frivolous, and girlish to take my mind off stress, like shopping." Marcia Israel often goes to a movie to unwind. "If you can totally identify with a character, you get out of yourself," she says.

Perfectionism is a self-induced stressor that plagues a lot of people and Debbi Fields is one of its victims. "Every time I do something average, I know it," she admits. Being a perfectionist serves her well in knocking out fabulous cookies, but she has worked hard to remove perfectionism from her personal life. In fact, in the last few years, Debbi has developed a new personal priority: "Having fun with my family, not cleaning closets." Debbi seems to be doing well in curbing her perfectionism these days: It took her more than four years to unpack the boxes from their last move. "I used to be Miss Perfect, but no more," boasts Debbi. "If I'm stressed, I reach out to somebody—play with my kids, call my mom, just get in touch." (Debbi has the right idea—researchers have recently linked loneliness and isolation to mortality and disease.) And, once again, a strong marriage makes its statement for health and low stress. Debbi says, "My husband is my best friend. We spend a lot of time laughing."

Arthur Woelfle, CB emeritus of Kraft, meditates twice a day, in the morning and in the evening, and "draws on it during the day." Robert McCowan, Ashland Oil, unwinds by shouting and stomping at football games. He says, "It's good to get excited over trivial things." James Kinnear agrees with Rudyard Kipling: "Keep your head while those about you are losing theirs." Breeding orchids and hunting with his spaniels helps this CEO of Texaco "keep his head."

Others rely on massage, a soak in a hot tub, a walk around the block, prayer, a few minutes alone, or just getting away from it all. Lucky Stores CEO, Larry DelSanto, thinks you should build a good support system around you in the business world and at home. "Don't try to do it alone," he advises. Larry's biggest supporter is his wife. Emmett Smith of LTV says he doesn't spend a lot of time worrying about worrying: "We raised four kids—it keeps you looking forward."

Robert Lundeen, former CB of Dow Chemical, says he learned the necessity of "getting away from it all," to maintain freshness and balance at the age of 42, when he was working in Hong Kong. After many frustrating weekends interrupted by business calls and on-the-spot meetings, he used a little creative thinking to come up with the perfect escape—sailing his yacht all day long every Sunday "with no phone on board."

Since most of us probably don't have a yacht docked in our backyard, we may have to settle for an inner tube in the city pool for

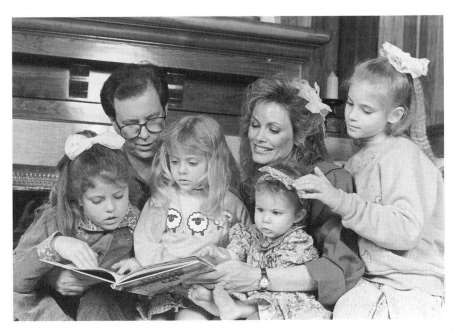

Bonds with husband and children are essential parts of Debbi Fields' HealthStyle. With Debbi and husband Randy is her own "in-home fitness program": five very active girls, four pictured here.

now. The point is that we can reap Lundeen's results ourselves with the proper perspective and a little imagination. We must take stress seriously and learn to handle it when it is present, as well as find ways to completely change the scenery at times. And by learning to refuel with Indy 500 efficiency, we can get optimal mileage out of a well-deserved break.

MENTAL FITNESS, ENDORPHINS, AND SUCCESS

In understanding how to beat stress, you should know a little about your own built-in anti-stressors: endorphins. Endorphins are proteins found in the brain, spinal cord, and endocrine glands. They are similar to opium derivatives such as morphine and are a natural painkiller, mood elevator, and tranquilizer all in one. They are said to affect sexual function, memory, and body temperature. Endorphins are responsible for creating the good feeling that was first associated with vigorous exercise, called the runner's high. Interestingly, the good feeling one feels after a hot Jacuzzi (especially followed by a cold shower) is also credited to a release of endorphins. Dow Chemical's CEO, Paul Oreffice, knows the effects of the endorphins. After landing in yet another hotel room after a long flight, heavy traffic, and bad food, instead of having a cocktail or trying to sleep, Paul takes a hot shower followed by a 10-second to 30-second cold shower and emerges revitalized and ready for his first meeting. Try it the next time you feel stressed, sluggish, or depressed. The elevation of energy and mood level that you will feel are endorphins in action (not to mention that your mood is bound to improve just by turning off the cold water).

Since endorphins are said to be released when we laugh (even the act of smiling is said to improve body chemistry) and when we help others, they are probably also released when we are doing anything we enjoy, such as a job to which we are well-suited. You can see how a nice little antistress endorphin cycle is perpetuated: loving what you do releases endorphins, endorphins enhance physical and mental energy and thus creativity, creativity releases more endorphins, and so on. More good news: the same basic things that produce endorphins boost the immune system. Good (endorphin) feelings create a healthy emotional state, and it is now believed that a healthy emotional state is related to a strong immune system. Research participants who practiced relaxation techniques once a day for three weeks had significantly fewer colds. Stay stress-free and you may stay cold-free.

THE ZEN OF SUCCESS: LIKE WHAT YOU DO

> Because I genuinely love what I do, my stress
> tends to be so much less. You don't pursue money,
> you pursue *love*.
>
> —Debbi Fields, CEO, President, Mrs. Fields' Cookies

"I never worried much about being successful," says James Kinnear, CEO of Texaco. "I was doing something I enjoyed, happened to be good at it, and success just came." The same story is repeated by others at the top. They just looked up from what they were doing one day and found themselves there. Robert McCowan of Ashland Oil advises young people accordingly: "Concentrate on what you're doing, not where you're going."

We can all relate to this to some extent. Most of us have had an interest, hobby, or sport that has consumed our whole attention—

made time disappear and given us a "high." Imagine this enthusiasm applied to your job. Common sense says you will be more successful at something you love doing, because, chances are, you are good at it. Not liking what you do depletes your vital energy and thus diminishes your chances for success.

Unfortunately, more than 90 percent of us are *not* satisfied with what we do. In contrast, the leaders in this book seem to have connected with their work in a way that complements their inner nature. They are at least partially self-actualized, to use psychological terminology. And that is the piece of the success puzzle that most of us are still missing.

A study of 1,500 top achievers found that the upper crust like the details of their jobs and are absorbed and motivated. They keep their minds on their activity (the work in front of them) rather than on the outcome (making money). They aren't competitive in the usual sense of trying to beat other people. They do, however, have strong personal goals and set high standards for themselves. To quote Rocky Johnson, CEO and chairman of GTE: "Aspiring is good for you."

The majority of the successes in my study have gotten where they are by following their hearts rather than the current money-making trend. They put their energy into doing their work well instead of focusing their attention on achieving specific advances. They concentrated on their own unique interests and talents, rather than trying to tailor their career to success. Once, in trying to evoke a response from an apathetic client in regard to career possibilities, I blurted, "Think hard. Is there *any*thing you like to do? Anything at all? Do you like to chew gum?" Silly as it may sound, this "pin yourself down" type of interrogation can be beneficial. Reduce your interests down to the simplest element. Don't think about geography, money, or logistics when answering the "What do you like to do" question.

Focus is the Key.   *Focus* is what happens when you are completely enamored with what you are doing. Focus is a concentrated connectedness that keeps you centered in the moment, instead of in the distracted (and most likely stressed) past or future. One CEO commented, "Barriers occur when you lose your focus, when you forget your priorities." Focus allows you to flow with the work process in a spontaneous, intuitive way, like a skilled athlete who performs a feat almost effortlessly. The interesting thing is that it doesn't seem to matter whether or not you have this esoteric understanding of your relationship to work. Neither does an athlete need to understand exactly which muscles he or she uses to get across the finish line. It just works and the athlete knows it. When you push yourself to your limits (creative, athletic, or otherwise), you make this connection and most probably do quite well with whatever is your object of focus. (It may be that exercise plays such an important part in the lives of these accomplished people, because exercise, like focus and creativity, has the capacity to bring you closer to self.)

I suspect most people who are successful first discover the connection with self through their connection with work, but the easier route for most of us may be to first become connected with self—then watch the connectedness with work and world follow closely behind. Some golfers are naturals, and others have had to study every aspect of the stroke—but both can shoot par.

One proven method of connecting with self and developing focus that extends beyond exercise is meditation. Some of the HWW leaders use formal meditation techniques, while I would guess many others are "naturals." The meditation technique that is outlined in the Mental Fitness Program (vipassana) is non-denominational and can be used solely as a stress management technique. It can also enhance your current religious preference (meditation is actually inherent in the history of most religions), or it can connect you to the "God within." In any case, the rewards are numerous: self-knowledge, higher consciousness, peace of mind, spiritual development, improved concentration, and, most probably, increased *success* in whatever you do. Focus seems to slow down the pace of life and put things in perspective, and without it you will remain distracted, disconnected, and stressed. Master the fine art of focus and you will discover a keener sense of awareness and a new sense of equanimity with the rest of the world.

A word about workaholism. Debbi Fields says it quite simply: "I'm a loveaholic, not a workaholic." A workaholic is a whole different animal. He or she is usually driven to work by fear, aggression, or alienation from family and society. Work allows the workaholic a place to escape or perhaps legitimize his or her existence. It is escapism, not inner connectedness. Work controls the workaholic. Unlike the workaholics, the people in this book are not only connected to their work and themselves (body and mind), but they are connected to the outside world around them, including community work, fitness, education of children, and helping individuals within their companies. In fact, when asked about their hobbies, many mentioned motivating and developing the skills of others as a genuine interest.

IS YOUR STRESS "POSITIVE" OR NEGATIVE?

Are you a stress hater or a stress lover? A recent study defined stress haters as goal-oriented, serious, and happiest without pressure.

Stress lovers were described as thriving on spontaneity and excitement and loving the thrill of the deadline.

The majority of the people in my study view problems as challenges, and pressure actually seems to fuel their motivation. Warren Batts, president emeritus of Dart & Kraft, likes solving problems so much that he considers problem-solving his creative outlet. Some of the CEOs confessed they overeat only when they get bored, and most say they are happiest when they are busy and involved. In fact, lack of stimulus—boredom—represents more of a stressor to them than high-pressure business transactions do. Judy's founder, Marcia Israel, agrees. "The only time I run out of energy is when I'm not busy," she says. "I'm fatigued when I'm discouraged or bored." Straddling the stimulus/boredom line can be a fine art for some. "My wife says I have a very thin window between boredom and exhaustion," admits Dr. Bob Boni, retired CEO of Armco. "I was retired for one month," says Mary Kay, head of Mary Kay Cosmetics, "and it was the worst month of my life. Every day, I read the obituaries to see if I was in them."

While I have a problem labeling *any* kind of stress as "positive," and, in fact, address this issue in my book *Conquering Stress*, there is no purpose in belaboring the point here. The bottom line is that the people I studied seem to thrive on what others would perceive as stress. With practice you can learn to experience stress in much the same way. The first step is to become familiar with the different types of stress.

Negative Stress

There are two categories of negative stress:

1. COGNITIVE STRESS.

With cognitive stress, you are quite aware of being stressed, and you resist it. You have no stress-reducing skills, so fear wraps around the stress, causing a snowball effect, that is, more stress. The solution? Mental Fitness techniques (to follow).

2. NON-COGNITIVE STRESS.

> You have to first recognize stress before you can take care of it. Stay in touch with yourself and don't turn your back on stress.
>
> —Gilda Marx, CEO, Gilda Marx Industries

With non-cognitive stress, you are not consciously aware of being stressed. You have "shoved it under the carpet" and are out of touch with your body and its reactions to some degree. You usually don't know when enough is enough and you keep pushing yourself. Small stressors are especially ignored. (In fact, studies show that small annoyances such as getting stuck in traffic or gaining a few pounds often have a greater impact on your health than do large-scale traumas, especially when the pressure is already high. So there's one more reason to lose weight—to reduce stress!

Non-cognitive stress is dangerous because it can sneak up from behind and hit you over the head with a heart attack or crippling back pain, to name two common problems. Learn to pay attention to the slow muscle tension build-up that signals stress. Become more aware of your body. Are you clenching your jaw, tensing your shoulders and back, or breathing shallowly? Take a moment to relax your body, take a few deep breaths or do a few stretches at your desk.

The Mental Fitness Program will help you establish your own stress management program and track your progress. Just five to twenty minutes a day of a relaxation program, even one you come up with yourself, can be significantly beneficial. If you have trouble learning the techniques, can't seem to tell if your body is relaxed or not, or would just like some "scientific" guidance, you can try biofeedback. A few biofeedback sessions can teach you how to release tension in every muscle group, and many health insurance policies will cover it.

"Positive" Stress

Work is more fun than fun.

—Mary Kay Ash quoting Edison

Mary Kay Ash of Mary Kay Cosmetics advises, "If you really want to get somewhere in a corporate operation, don't look at the clock and worry about whether it's time to quit." That is good advice for anyone who is unfamiliar with being fully immersed in his or her work, which makes checking the clock redundant. The person who experiences pressure as a challenge might work fast but usually doesn't feel rushed or stressed. There is a certain inner quietness. He or she just seems to see and feel things at a slower pace.

How can you do this? With a focus technique I call Visual Slow Down. I incorporated this technique from something I learned during a tennis match several years ago. Reid, my doubles partner (and superior player) approached me for a little midgame powwow (we were losing). He told me that I have more time than I think to hit what I categorized as "bullet balls" that were flying past me at the net. He told me to concentrate on nothing but the ball as it approached; to watch it and slow it down with my eyes, rather than reacting with my usual panicked, scattered response. I was desperate and didn't have time to analyze his theory—I just did it. And it worked! The world seemed to freeze while the ball almost floated through the air as if in slow-motion, like an overproduced TV commercial. It actually seemed as if I slowed down time. Later, I realized that the same principle works outside the court. Example: You are stressed and things seem to be moving at triple speed—cars racing by, hectic office pace, and so forth. You simply pick one object (such as one "racing" car), concentrate on it, and s l o w   i t   d o w n with your eyes. Do it a few more times. You should soon see a slower world in front of you versus one stressful blur. You can still hurry, but you needn't get tangled up in the race. Just watch it, and slow it down. Use the Mental Fitness Calendar to chart your practice.

HOW DO YOU REACT TO STRESS?

> If you don't have health, it is difficult to operate in a high-stress environment.
>
> —Dr. Bob Boni, CEO emeritus, Armco

To fully employ the Mental Fitness Program, you need to examine your reaction to stress, so you can begin to restructure your response accordingly.

I have previously discussed Type A and Type B personalities and I now want you to assess your own personality. This rather basic A/B differentiation of personalities allows you a useful way to identify yourself, and troubleshoot accordingly.

Are You a Type A?   A line from a James Taylor song perhaps best describes the inner drivenness of the Type A personality: "It hurts my motor to go so slow . . ."* Type A's seem to have their carburetors set just a little bit higher than others. This commonly manifests itself with a sense of time urgency and competitiveness, often accompanied by an underlying or overt anger or hostility. Chronic hostility and anger can be bad for your health, since they have been linked to heart disease. In fact, according to Dr. Redford Williams at Duke University, those with high hostility at age 19 tend to have high cholesterol when they are 40. In any case, if you have any of these traits, you may be the faster paced (Type A) variety. If you are relaxed, even-tempered, patient, a good listener, and a slow and deliberate speaker, you are probably a Type B, and you may handle stress fairly well already.

---

*"Traffic Jam" by James Taylor. Copyright © 1977 Country Road Music, Inc. (BMI). All rights reserved. Used by permission.

If you recognize Type A behavior in yourself (and 75 percent of American city dwellers should), don't worry—there's hope. Beatrice's CEO emeritus, Fred Rentschler, is living proof. Fred used to be a full-fledged Type A but says he is almost a certified Type B now. "I have been working more now towards getting a lower handicap and getting better at fishing. For the first time, I'm really setting goals that are more to recreate, that include greater quantities of rose-smelling rather than an occasional sniff on the fast track."

"Go with the flow" is a Sixties phrase that aptly describes how to deal with stress. I prefer an even older formula: Suffering equals Pain multiplied by Resistance (or, S = P × R). Resistance is what causes suffering and stress. Stop resisting and your suffering will also stop (see meditation techniques, Chapter 8). Pain, or stress, may still be present, but it will be experienced in a nonsuffering, often insightful, way. As stress expert Hans Seyle discovered: Stress is merely what you perceive it to be. In other words, much of your stress is essentially of your own making. That thought may be a little unsettling, but don't let it cause you more stress.

Learn to take life's laps at your own pace. "I have to come first," says Gilda Marx. "I can be a loving, creative, energetic person, a good mother, wife, business person, companion and partner, but not if I deny myself. If I take care of me, I can take care of the world around me."

TIPS
TO REMEMBER

- *The successful people I studied prioritize stress management and handle stress well.*
- *They have been married 22-1/2 years longer than the average American.*
- *You will feel less stress if you have a positive perspective, a sense of humor, a personal interest and commitment to your work, a feeling of challenge and a sense of control over your life.*

BE
RELENTLESSLY
PATIENT

Chapter Eight

The
Healthy, Wealthy,
& Wise Mental
Fitness Program

Many different stress management techniques and tricks have already been mentioned. A few more are described here in the Mental Fitness Program. Find the one(s) that work for you and commit to them. These techniques will help you reduce stress and develop a better attitude, whether you are a Type A or Type B, a stress lover or a stress hater.

An added bonus: Besides reducing stress and tension, stress management techniques also provide benefits in other areas. According to a study in which stress management techniques were taught in several major industrial companies, the following benefits were reported:

1. Increased clarity of thinking
2. Better concentration

(See the back of the book for guided meditation/stress management audio tapes or make your own from the descriptions that follow.)

3. Improved self-esteem

4. Improved creativity

5. Improved job satisfaction

6. Decreased irritability, anger, anxiety

7. Decreased job turnover

The Mental Fitness Program can be the most fun part of your efforts to improve your HealthStyle. After all, building your mental fitness requires no sweat or hunger pangs! But do give proper attention to it because without mental fitness, the benefits of your diet and exercise programs may be limited. Descriptions of eight types of stress reducers follow. The Mental Fitness Calendar follows the discussion of these stress reducers.

EIGHT WAYS TO REDUCE STRESS AND IMPROVE YOUR MENTAL FITNESS

In the descriptions that follow, much attention is placed on the first technique, Meditation/Relaxation. It requires a bit more explanation, and I believe it is an invaluable component of any successful program. As meditation teacher Shinzen Young says, "meditation is to the mind what exercise is to the body."

1. Meditation/Relaxation Techniques

I was surprised to learn how many of America's most powerful leaders either meditate or have tried it. Studies show that meditation lowers blood pressure and cholesterol. One reason for this may be that meditation offers true contentment and relaxation. It probably doesn't surprise you to know that we are seldom completely relaxed. Even when asleep, we contract muscles and grind our teeth and often wake up feeling worse than when we went to bed.

Meditation also enables us to master complete focus, the ability to stay in the *now*. If you think about it, we are seldom completely in the present. Most of us bustle along, reliving the past or preoccupied with the future, until we wake up one day and realize that our life is almost over, and it seems we somehow missed the show.

Zen masters speak of experiencing everything fully. The classic example is that of meditating while washing the dishes. The idea is not to think of being *done* with the task but of being *one* with it— entering a state of timelessness and complete concentration. Fully experience the warmth of the water on your hands, the hardness of the plate, the softness of the sponge, and so forth. Before you know it, the dishes are done and you are floating in tranquility rather than exhaustion. As you practice, you will become more skilled and your entire life will be affected—including your work. Meditation serves the same purpose as practicing scales on the piano so that you are able to play the song. The "scales" of meditation result in experiencing the present more fully and enjoying a higher quality life.

Choose the following meditation technique(s) that suits your personality. While entire books (including my book, *Conquering Stress)* have been devoted to the subject of stress, I have chosen the techniques that, in my experience, are most effective and easily applicable. In addition to these techniques, feel free to experiment—take classes, listen to tapes, read. Find the method that works best for you. To ensure your success, be patient and make a time commitment on your Mental Fitness Calendar or on any other calendar. As with diet and exercise, you will have your good and bad days, weeks, and even months.

Stick with your meditation practice and don't let life's hamster wheel tempt you to skip or shorten your sessions, rushing you off to yet another of life's endless errands. For many busy, successful people, sitting completely still for even five minutes can initially seem an impossible task. What? No phone calls? No meetings? However, once experienced in full, meditation is quickly viewed as an invaluable investment of time, a refueling.

Vipassana Meditation (Insight Meditation). Vipassana meditation is perhaps one of the least-known but most effective meditation techniques around. Vipassana is an age-old body scanning technique that acts as your personal biofeedback monitor—at no cost. Unlike some other techniques that are solely relaxation-oriented, vipassana meditation goes deeper, breaking up knots of the past that manifest in personality through cravings (including addictions) and aversions (avoidances). In breaking up these deep-seated character defects, the all-too-familiar condition called suffering diminishes. Vipassana teaches us how to experience suffering (physical, mental, emotional) in a new, self-freeing way. Thomas Merton once said that he didn't become a monk to suffer more than others, but to suffer more *effectively* than others. Fortunately, "monkdom" is not a necessary step in freeing ourselves from suffering. Vipassana meditation effects permanent transformation while developing body-mind awareness, a deeper state of spiritual connection, and a softer understanding of the world.

In a sense, this practice is merely a condensed replica of real life. For most of us, life is a series of stimulations and distractions which we use to run from one reality or another (responsibilities, loneliness, age, time, self). This running is precisely where addictions are born—

whether it's shopping, eating, or alcoholism. We are overstimulated, and we keep ourselves that way so we don't have to feel what ultimate stillness and solitude bring. We subconsciously fear it will be a lonely, dark void, when it, in fact, is the opposite. By putting yourself in the sensorially deprived atmosphere of meditation, you are forced to stop and look at (and dissolve) your demons (in the form of negative body sensations) head-on. A rarity for most of us. When was the last time you sat quietly alone, without distraction? (Incidentally, some forward-thinking psychologists are now using vipassana to help patients make the connection between mind, body, and emotions.)

To practice vipassana meditation, get into a comfortable sitting or lying position, spine straight, eyes closed. Many of my MCA/ Universal clients prefer to lie on the carpet with feet up, since they sit behind desks most of the day. This is acceptable as long as you don't fall asleep. Try to remain motionless for the next ten to thirty minutes (five to ten at the start is fine).

One vipassana technique is called *noting*. Carefully tune into the spot or area in your body with the most prominent sensation. Feel everything that's going on—to the core. Keep noting the area, out loud or silently, as you study it. "Forehead. Forehead. Forehead." Identify the exact region of the sensation. Draw an imaginary circle around it. Be aware of every sensation within the circle and feel each to the fullest, with absolutely no resistance. Just watch the area and allow the tension or pain to melt away. What starts as a glacier—a mountain of solid ice—becomes an ice cube, then a puddle. Stay with one area until the ice cube is "melted" and then stare at the puddle of tranquility for a moment. Then move on to another prominent sensation and repeat the process. If you feel the urge to shift positions, scratch, or think of something you "have" to do, resist the temptation. That is just your tricky subconscious trying to run from the homework at hand. Ride it as you would a bucking bronco—and stay with it. You will be amazed at how stress will melt away with bodily tensions.

A more methodical system of using vipassana is to *scan* top to bottom, bottom to top. This system can be used exclusively or when you don't have any blatant issues or bodily tensions or pains to address. Start at the head and slowly scan down to the feet, feeling every inch along the way (feel your skin against your clothes or just "existing"; go deeper and feel your muscles and even your organs as you get more advanced). "Look" at each area as if you've never felt it before; as if this is a fascinating discovery (it is—think of your body as your own personal TV screen). I often ask clients to feel this scan as a "rolling pin of awareness" passing over the body. Start with the forehead and fully feel it from top to bottom (taking 30 to 60 seconds). Then, move into the eye area and observe the tension you

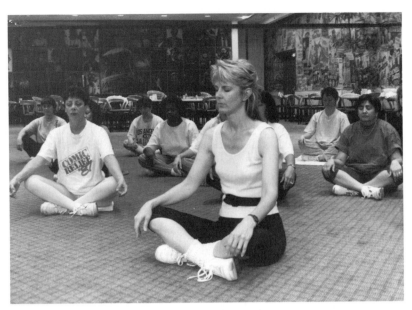

KRS teaching stress management at MCA/Universal.

probably weren't even aware that you held in your eyelids and corners of the eyes. Notice the relaxing take place as you bring awareness to each area (try this right now).

Next, move to the jaw muscles and feel the tension melt away (these muscles are tight on a lot of people and are often said to be where anger is lodged). Move slowly down the cheeks to the mouth, throat and neck, chest, diaphragm, stomach, lower abdomen, thighs, knees, calves, ankles, and feet. Then reverse the process, scanning back up to the head, staying in the state of complete awareness of sensation. If you have trouble staying focused, talk aloud—"Forehead [pause] eyelids [pause], jaw [pause]," etc. The whole process should take about 20 minutes. This technique is relaxing but is also self-educating. It imparts full meaning to the expression "listen to your body."

Daily meditation will make you, in the words of vipassana teacher Shinzen Young, "internally literate" and capable of identifying and eliminating stress at its inception. For example, as you are running late for an appointment, you will be able to spot when and where tension is building and diffuse it "in action," arriving at your destination with nerves intact.

Two nice side benefits of vipassana meditation are heightened mental and physical sensitivity and awareness. Be sure to *slow down* enough to experience and appreciate them. For example, notice the cozy texture of your sock against your skin as you snuggle it on. Feel the cool smoothness of the sheets as you slip into bed at night. Experience the joy of a puppy at play. Hear the music of water boiling on the stove. See the poetry in a soaring jet, as if through a photographer's lens.

I suggest choosing one simple activity on which you will focus full awareness (such as washing your face in the evening or eating at least one bite of food very slowly with awareness—perhaps the first bite—of one, two, or three meals a day). Move in slow motion, noting every sensation you feel in your body as you go ("Hand. Lips. Tongue. Roof of Mouth. Throat."). Chart your goals and progress on the Mental Fitness Calendar that follows. Gradually add activities of focused awareness.

Word/Object Meditation.   This meditation technique uses a word (mantra) or an object (such as a candle) as its focus of concentration. The mantra can be meaningful or meaningless (Herbert Benson suggests the word *one* in *The Relaxation Response*). For some people this technique is a good one to start with before moving on to other techniques, such as vipassana, while others stay with it for a lifetime. Some of the CEOs I studied use TM (transcendental meditation), which is a word/mantra repetition. It brings a calm, blissful state quite easily while developing concentration.

To practice word/object meditation, get comfortably seated, eyes closed (unless focusing on an object), and concentrate solely and completely on the object or word for ten to thirty minutes. That's all there is to it. There is no mind-altering voodoo going on here—the idea is to give the childlike mind something to focus on, since its inclination is to run wild from thought to thought. Some teachers call it the "monkey mind." One ancient "yoga joke" depicts a master telling his students that if he had a dog he would name it Mind. He could then train it: "Sit Mind, fetch Mind, be still Mind . . ." (Not a real laugher, but that's yoga humor for you.)

So, when the monkey mind wanders during meditation (and it will), simply and gently return to your word/object of focus. After the first few antsy minutes of settling down, you'll notice a calm that beats a glass of wine and can compete with a trip to the Bahamas.

Breath Awareness Meditation.   This technique is essentially the same as Word/Object Focus, but deserves special mention and instruction. Breath awareness is similarly excellent on its own or as a warm-up to other techniques, such as vipassana.

To practice breath awareness meditation, sit comfortably with eyes closed. Focus your attention on the breath at the base of the nostrils (above the lip), feeling the air enter and exit through the nose.

Some people feel the air better at the back or upper part of the throat, and others like to focus on the movement of the diaphragm. Take your pick and then stay with it. This technique doesn't give the mind a lot to do, so while it is eventually wonderful for quieting the mind and developing concentration, the mind will initially want to keep running to its playground of thoughts. Quietly bring your mind back "by the hand"—with no scoldings (frustration or guilt).

Contraction-Release Relaxation.   To use the contraction-release relaxation technique, lie down with eyes closed. Start with the feet and move your way up to the head: Tense the toes (isolating just the toes), hold for five to ten seconds and relax for five to ten seconds. Tense the feet, relax. Move to the calves, thighs, buttocks, stomach, torso, arms, face, and finally the whole body, tensing and releasing. This will not only give you a wonderfully relaxed sensation but will also help you be aware of what tension is, where it is, and how it is released. Most people go to their graves never having really relaxed. In fact, if you've ever seen a person die, you'll notice that within about 15 minutes, they are almost unrecognizable. The tension leaves the body and with it many of the wrinkles that are held by a lifetime of resistance (remember, Suffering = Pain × Resistance).

Head-to-Toe Relaxation.   This relaxation method is the same basic approach as the contraction-release method, except that you skip the tensing part. In other words, you just relax each part of the body, from the head down (or from the feet up). It is perfect for insomnia, since most people don't make it halfway through before falling asleep. If you want to stay awake, do the exercise sitting or even standing. This relaxation can be done with soft music.

Visualization Meditation.   Visualization meditation is a multi-faceted technique that is invaluable. Among other things, this technique can be used to relax, or to enhance self-healing, self-image, or athleticism (this technique is popular among world-class athletes). You relax for about five minutes (using any of the techniques described previously) while lying, sitting, or standing. You then bring up a picture in your mind of what you are trying to accomplish. Once you master some favorite visualizations, you can bring up powerful 1 to 10-second versions of them throughout your busy day.

> (1) Relaxation: You can visualize going somewhere (a mini-vacation) imagined or real, such as that mountain stream where you love to fish, or back to relive your last vacation. Perhaps you'd rather just see yourself falling backwards into a puff of clouds, releasing your tight grasp of the

world and surrendering to serenity for a few precious moments. Or you can picture a stream flowing through your body, up and down, flushing out tension as it gushes through. Just feel the energy releasing as the cleansing takes place.

(2) Athleticism and Self-Image: Another effective application is to visualize yourself as the person you want to be—athletically, mentally, spiritually, financially, and so forth. Picture yourself; see what you are wearing, where you are (an English country road with the sun pouring down through the trees), how you feel, and the look on your face. Become that picture.

(3) Self-Healing: Visualization can also be used to enhance healing. Many people have had success in lowering their blood pressure, curing migraines, healing ulcers and just about everything else imaginable, including heart disease and cancer, by using visualization. There has even been some impressive work done with slowing of the AIDS virus. Visualization obviously doesn't preclude proper medical attention. Many have tried this approach when conventional medicine has failed, however, and have had success. In this form of visualization, you begin with five minutes of any of the above techniques, such as Breath Awareness or Head-to-Toe Relaxation. Then visualize the area of sickness or disease being infiltrated by "goodness" for five to twenty minutes. It's nice if you can choose your own "goodness" image, but some have pictured the warm healing rays of the sun coming in and "zapping" the area, much like laser beams. Others like to picture a good army entering the area to kill off the bad guys (disease germs). Experiment.

2. Learn How to Breathe

Breathing is something we do about 20,000 times a day. When we are stressed, our breathing becomes rapid, shallow, and often "paradoxical." Paradoxical breathers breathe "backwards." This means they fill their upper lungs first, lower portions second. Breathing experts says this type of breathing causes more stress. Thus, the stress cycle is perpetuated. Shallow breathers fill only the top portion of their lungs and don't exhale fully. This means more residual carbon dioxide in the lungs and less oxygen to the brain and muscles, which contributes to mental and physical lethargy. Toxic irritants build up that can lead to infections and disease. Average lungs can expand to volume of almost 6,000 cubic centimeters. Unfortunately, we normally use only 600 to 700 cubic centimeters. And smog doesn't help matters. City dwellers commonly test below average on Peak Flow breath tests. Breathing exercises can restore proper breathing skills and emotional equanimity, as well as help offset diminishing lung capacity and strength, whether from smog, stress, or age. Breathing exercises can also provide an immediate energy boost (increased oxygen) or can act as an on-the-spot stress and pain reducer. Deep breathing may be such a good stress fighter because it is said to release endorphins that, as you remember, are our bodies' natural tranquilizer. Similarly, breathing reduces pain, as endorphins are also our bodies' natural pain killer. That's one of the reasons breathing works so well in natural childbirth. Chart your Breathing Exercises plan on your Mental Fitness Calendar at the end of this chapter.

Baby's Breath.   To witness proper breathing firsthand, watch a baby sleeping. See the whole torso expand and contract freely and completely. Lie on your stomach with your arms in a comfortable position. Let yourself sink into the floor or bed and relax. Use soft music or a few minutes of the aforementioned meditation techniques. As you relax, notice your breathing getting deeper. Feel your diaphragm/navel area expanding and releasing. Then feel your whole body "breathing." Stay with it for about five minutes, appreciating and memorizing the feel of proper breathing. Then slowly roll over onto your back and continue for another five minutes. This position is just slightly more "advanced." Put your hand over your diaphragm/navel area and feel your body's natural breathing rhythm and capacity. Don't try to control or force the breathing process—just let the breath do its own thing.

Then slowly sit up and do the same. It might help to have your eyes closed. Keep your concentration on your Baby's Breath. As you get more advanced, you can try standing and eventually walking while you continue this exercise. The idea is to be doing this breathing all the time, including when you are stressed. For the first few weeks, you may want to stay with the stomach position only and work into the other positions as you feel ready. Indicate your plan on the Mental Fitness Calendar.

Complete Breath.   The Complete Breath increases lung capacity and can bring immediate stress relief at your desk, in your car, or standing in lines. This exercise is done to the count of 12 (inhalation) and 8 (exhalation). Both inhalation and exhalation are long and slow. You want to feel as if you are "stretching" your lungs on the inhalation, as if you are filling a balloon.

First, exhale completely, eliminating every bit of air. Then slowly start to inhale through your nose, filling the lower portion of your lungs/diaphragm area first (four counts), your middle portion/ rib cage area next (four counts), and your upper lobes/upper chest area last (four counts). This totals twelve counts. Now hold the breath for eight counts and feel the expansion of the lungs. Then exhale through the mouth or nose slowly, in reverse—from top of lungs to bottom (eight to twelve counts). Doing this exercise once may be enough to reduce much of your stress, but repeat several times to establish the habit of proper breathing.

Breath of Fire.   This is a Kundalini yoga exercise that is said to increase energy and lung capacity, cleanse the blood, and eliminate old toxins from the lungs. An added bonus: It helps tone the stomach. The best way to describe Breath of Fire is to tell you to pant like a dog on a hot day—fast and hard. Instead of mouth breathing with tongue hanging out, however, use only your nose—for inhalations as well as exhalations. Another helpful description is to think of the exhalation as if you were getting punched in the stomach and having the wind knocked out of you. The moving part is the diaphragm, not the chest. In a sitting or standing position, put your hand on your diaphragm/navel area and begin to "nose pant" to the count of 10 to start, giving yourself approximately 1 second per "pant." Many people have trouble controlling this muscle and need to start more slowly and concentrate a little harder at first. As you get more proficient, extend your count and speed. Do several rounds—Breath of Fire for 30 seconds, rest for 15 to 30 seconds, and so forth. Students of Kundalini yoga commonly alternate between 3 to 20 minutes of Breath of Fire with 2 minutes of rest, and repeat this pattern 5 times. Count yourself lucky—you needn't get that enthusiastic to gain results. If you feel any dizziness at first, stop and take it a little slower. With practice, you will build fast and will feel no dizziness.

3. Give of Yourself

Helping others has been shown to reduce stress and is something for which the executives in my study make time. At least once a day, do one little thing for someone else with no thought of reward or recognition. Just a smile at someone passing will do for starters.

4. Laugh

Rent funny videos (and keep an emergency private stock), watch funny TV shows, read funny books, or start your own "funny book" of incidents and jokes you collect from daily life (my favorite laugh source). Most important, don't take life so seriously and do learn to laugh at yourself. Laughter is healing. Let me try to fill your daily quota. Old joke (a warning for those of you who don't like scripted humor): Don't try to teach a rabbit to tap dance. It wastes your time and annoys the rabbit.

It is probably no coincidence that most of the low-stress HWW leaders have a great sense of humor (the interviews for this book were laced with laughs). Humor, after all, is an effective stress antidote— it helps keep things in perspective. Studies show that the presence of positive factors (such as humor) is more important than the lack of negative factors in reducing stress. Laughter aids circulation, releases endorphins, massages stomach muscles, stimulates digestion, lowers blood pressure, enhances respiration, and oxygenates your blood. Studies have shown that laughter reduces stress just as effectively as biofeedback does.

5. Nurture Friendships—Furry or Otherwise

Set aside a specific time each week for family or friends you are comfortable with and share your joys as well as your troubles (this is a good practice for men, often considered less emotionally open than women). Again, many of the executives, male and female alike, mentioned talking and/or walking with their mate as a form of stress reduction.

Also, seriously consider acquiring a pet. Experts have found that just about any pet, including fish and birds, can be considered man's best friend. Many of the executives mentioned playing with or walking with their dogs as a stress reducer. Pets can reduce stress, lower blood pressure, get owners motivated to exercise (a dog more so than a fish), and generally give owners a sense of well-being. Pets now are being used effectively in retirement homes as a means of providing love and purpose to lonely elderly persons. Do a good deed too and get your pet from the local pound!

6. Adjust Your Attitude

Choose one area of your life in which you are going to practice being more positive and optimistic. Write it on your Mental Fitness Calendar and consciously work on it each day. Catch yourself whenever that negative "can't do" attitude sneaks in. Example: Practice enjoying your present career status instead of dwelling on your future aspirations, which can lead to stress and unhappiness. Another application: If you are a negative thinker and know it, write down one positive thing about your day each night of the first week, two things each night the second week, and so forth up to five (or more) things. You will soon start thinking more positively, if only to collect your daily quota of "five positive things."

Also, acquire an appreciation of life *now*. In speaking of the passage of time, Paul McCartney recently expressed this concept quite plainly: *"Now* is never very important to most people ... but it's really all we've got." I often suggest trying to maintain a "near-death" appreciation of life. By this, I mean that "just glad to be alive" feeling we've all had after being very sick. For the first day or two of recovery, you suddenly appreciate otherwise insignificant things (such as the feeling of fresh air blowing across your face or even seeing the crabby old man next door) and soak everything in as if for the first—or *last*—time. Work at getting that feeling into every moment of every day.

7. Practice Type-A Drills

First, learn to recognize when you are in the midst of rushed, driven behavior. Make a commitment to eat, talk, drive, and move more slowly. Be patient. Enjoy the process (of life). Listen. Start a creative hobby, learn to laugh at yourself, learn to "do nothing" well, write letters, write about stress—what is causing you stress and how you might remedy it. (Just writing about stress has been shown to increase white blood cell count, which boosts the immune system.) Become aware of facial and body movements and tics as well and your sense of time urgency (always rushing and feeling "behind".) Do not attempt to rationalize your (Type A) behavior, just commit to stopping it (don't listen to the arguments your "A" self gives to rationalize its compulsive behavior). Pick one of these skills at a time (if you're a car commuter, start with your attitudes and behavior when you're behind the wheel). You'll be surprised at how working on one area will quickly spread to other areas. It thus becomes unnecessary to tackle each item individually.

8. Have Fun

Most people are so caught up in the process of "life's stuff" that they forget how to have fun—even when they are allegedly having fun ("Darn it! I missed that putt by one inch. That puts me two over. What a lousy day!") Your new HWW HealthStyle Program is about adding fullness to your life, not just taking away the negative habits.

Cultivate a fun mentality and try to add fun to your life on a daily basis: Meet a friend for lunch. Play with the children or dog, kid around with co-workers, listen to music (like pets, music is one of life's therapeutic freebies). Get a massage, go dancing or to a movie, or, as one CEO suggested, learn to play a great game of poker. And take vacations. One- or two-day trips are great rejuvenators. Be spontaneous with fun, too, but don't rely on spontaneity for your fun "quota."

Note on your Mental Fitness Calendar (which follows) any specific fun you are resolving to incorporate into your HealthStyle.

YOUR HEALTHSTYLE RECORD-KEEPING

Keep Records to Keep Motivated

It's important that you make your HWW HealthStyle Program fit into your life rather than vice versa. Very few of us have the time, interest, or patience to stay with a demanding program, and we are consequently often left with feelings of failure and guilt, along with the pot belly with which we started. But you can eliminate this vicious cycle by tailoring your program to fit into your life and by keeping records, especially in the crucial beginning stages.

Charts and calendars are good tools to help you facilitate and measure your progress. They can help you coordinate and customize a program that is unique to you while remaining true to the examples you have read about. It is not absolutely necessary that you utilize these charts, however. Their purpose is to teach you skills and make things easier for you, not to create more work or stress. Some of my clients love this tool and, in fact, keep ongoing records, while others use it for just the first few months. Keep all of your HealthStyle records in a special envelope-type folder for easy reference and use.

Do realize, however, that there is a definite purpose in keeping daily records for at least 60 to 90 days. Remind yourself of this short timespan, that it doesn't have to be forever. Also remind yourself that the skills acquired during this period will serve you for a lifetime. These skills will help you stay on course and motivated when things seem toughest.

Feel free to reproduce and enlarge all of the charts and calendars so that you can use them as long as you like.

Your HWW Personal Goals Chart

Goals are a productive tool for any area of self-improvement. The following chart is provided for specific monthly goalmaking. It is particularly effective because you "report in" at the end of each month ("End Result"). (For daily recordkeeping of your monthly goals,

Your Personal Goals Chart

MONTH OF _____ GOALS / DIARY

	BEGINNING GOALS	END RESULTS
1. EXERCISE (time, activity, etc.)	Walk one mile three days a week	YES!
2. DIET (weight loss guidelines, calorie goals, fat reduced)		
3. NUTRITION (foods added, omitted)	Drink 2 glasses of water a day	25 days - yes
4. ALCOHOL		
5. TIME MANAGEMENT		
6. STRESS MANAGEMENT (relaxation, etc.)		
7. DRESS/SELF IMAGE		
8. WEIGHT	148	145
9. PLEASURES		
10. NOTES (changes, thoughts, additional accomplishments, etc.)		

(Chart your daily progress on the Diet & Exercise, HealthStyle, or Mental Fitness calendars.)

156

Your Personal Goals Chart

MONTH OF _____ GOALS / DIARY

BEGINNING GOALS	END RESULTS
1. <u>EXERCISE</u> (time, activity, etc.)	
2. <u>DIET</u> (weight loss guidelines, calorie goals, fat reduced)	
3. <u>NUTRITION</u> (foods added, omitted)	
4. <u>ALCOHOL</u>	
5. <u>TIME MANAGEMENT</u>	
6. <u>STRESS MANAGEMENT</u> (relaxation, etc.)	
7. <u>DRESS/SELF IMAGE</u>	
8. <u>WEIGHT</u>	
9. <u>PLEASURES</u>	
10. <u>NOTES</u> (changes, thoughts, additional accom-plishments, etc.)	

(Chart your daily progress on the Diet & Exercise, HealthStyle, or Mental Fitness calendars.)

use the HWW Diet and Exercise Calendar and/or the HWW HealthStyle Calendars that follow.) Save your Personal Goal Chart from month to month. This can be quite motivating, as progress can seem slow on a daily or even a monthly basis, but when viewed over a period of time the overall progress picture can be truly exciting.

How to Use Your Mental Fitness Calendar

The HWW Mental Fitness Calendar can help you acquire the same skills used by those in my study. Consistent with the HWW philosophy, the idea is to master just one or two (if easy) stress reducer(s) at a time. When you feel it is successfully incorporated into your life, you can add another one. It is beneficial to give each stress reducer at least 8 to 12 weeks before adding another. The most important thing is to track your progress until the habit is established in order to maintain your awareness and resolve. Decide when, where, and how often you will do these techniques and note it on the calendar provided. Copy this calendar and use it in conjunction with your Personal Goals Chart on page 156.

If you are working on "Friends" and decide you would like to get together with friends on Tuesdays and Fridays, circle *Friends*, *Tuesday*, *Friday* (and cross off the days as you complete them). In the "Time" column, write in the time of day for those stress reducers that require planning ahead. For example, in fulfilling your Laugh quota, you might prefer to schedule a specific night to rent a comedy video, rather than ordering yourself to "Laugh, 8 P.M. Friday" (that's a little joke). The point is that while this might sound a bit mechanical at first, it's how you establish habits. By the way, a good time for a shot of humor is just before going to sleep. Your state of mind at bedtime stays with you until morning. Why not wake up laughing? This is not as far-fetched as it may sound. I know people (myself included) who have awakened themselves laughing from a funny dream. It sure beats nightmares.

How to use your HWW Diet & Exercise Calendar

To help you accomplish your diet and exercise goals, use the following HWW Exercise Calendars to record your daily diet and/or exercise. Avoid becoming a chronic scale watcher, however. Chronic scale watching puts an unhealthy emphasis on the numbers. Weigh no more than once a week. To figure your calories to maintain or lose weight, see "A Failproof Formula for Losing Weight," page 209.

First, log your daily food intake and calories (cal.) of each food. Example: 1 apple 80 (cal.). (Tip: Keep a personal quickreference list of your most frequently eaten foods.) Total and circle your total caloric intake at the end of each day (bottom of Food Diary columns). Then, under Activity Diary, write down the calories you burned for the day based on Low, Medium, and High exercise activity. Low activity burns 3 calories per minute, Medium burns 5 calories per minute, and High burns 7 calories per minute. Example: Moderate walk—30 minutes—150 calories. Total and circle your daily exercise calories at the bottom of Activity Diary columns.

Add your daily totals at the end of each week and enter your weekly diet and exercise totals and daily average (divide total by 7). It's interesting to compare your totals week to week and see for yourself that it works. Don't skip a day or simply write "Bad Day." Most of the time people haven't done as badly as they think, and realizing this can resurrect morale. And if it's a truly bad day, facing reality is much healthier and less painful than running from it. Feel free to photocopy (and enlarge).

How to use your HWW HealthStyle Calendar— Psychological Record

If you opt to use the HWW Diet & Exercise Calendar, you may want to utilize the following calendar as a psychological record, to record any outstanding events of the day and how you felt physically and mentally. This record will help you spot reasons for relapse and enable you to permanently circumvent them. This method can be extremely valuable for revealing patterns not otherwise evident that could be undermining your program. (Example: May 4—"Didn't make deadlines at work. Ate sweets after dinner in front of TV.") From such entries, you might conclude that frustrations about your job make you overeat and that no job is worth making you fat.

Or, if you opt not to use the HWW Diet & Exercise Calendar or Mental Fitness Calendar, use the following HWW HealthStyle Calendar in the way that best suits you. For example, you can mark a big red X on each day that you complete your exercise, don't eat sugar, don't smoke or stay within your caloric guideline (write in calories if you wish)—whichever you are working on. If you want to track both, you might use two different markers—for example, an X for exercise completed and a gold star for good diet days. After you have accomplished these goals, you can use the same X method for tracking other goals (such as doing stretches or giving up caffeine).

The visual effect of this method is powerful and motivating. And if you feel a weak moment approaching, you can take a look at your progress. When you see ten Xs in a row, you'll say: "Why blow it now? I'm doing better than I thought. I want my X for the day." Feel free to photocopy (and enlarge).

Mental Fitness Calendar
Week of _Nov. 16_

Stress Reducer	Specific Goals and Time	Mon.	Tues.	Wed.	Thurs.	Fri.	Sat.	Sun.
Meditation/Relaxation								
Learn How to Breathe	The Complete Breath 8am - 5 min	✓	✓	✓	✓	✓	✓ (10a.m.)	✓ (10 a.m.)
Give of Yourself								
Nurture Friendships (Furry or Otherwise)								
Adjust Your Attitude	Write down 1 positive thing - bedtime	✓	✓	✓	✓	✓	✓	✓
Practice Type A Drills								
Have Fun								
Other Mental Fitness Goals								

Mental Fitness Calendar

Week of _____

Stress Reducer	Specific Goals and Time	Mon.	Tues.	Wed.	Thurs.	Fri.	Sat.	Sun.
Meditation/Relaxation								
Learn How to Breathe								
Give of Yourself								
Nurture Friendships (Furry or Otherwise)								
Adjust Your Attitude								
Practice Type A Drills								
Have Fun								
Other Mental Fitness Goals								

Diet & Exercise Calendar

Name _Sarah_

Week Beginning _January 1_

Daily Maintenance Calories _2220_ / Weekly _15.540_

Daily Calories to lose 2 lbs/week _1220_ / Weekly _8.540_

(Weekly = Daily x 7)

FOOD DIARY

Monday		Tuesday		Wednesday		Thursday		Friday		Saturday		Sunday	
Foods	Cal.	Foods	Cal.	Foods	Cal.	Foods	Cal.	Foods	Cal.	Foods	Cal.	Foods	Cal.
Cereal & Skim Milk	150												
	100												
Fruit													
Salad	300												
Roll	125												
Cookie	75												
Fish	150												
Potato & Broccoli	150												
Popcorn	150												
Total:	1200	Total:		Total:		Total:		Total:		Total:		Total:	

EXERCISE DIARY

Minutes	Cal.	Minutes	Cal.	Minutes	Cal.	Minutes	Cal.	Minutes	Cal.	Minutes	Cal.	Minutes	Cal.
30-min walk	180												
Total:	180	Total:		Total:		Total:		Total:		Total:		Total:	

Light Activity: 3 cal/min Medium Activity: 5 cal/min Heavy Activity: 7 cal/min

TOTAL FOOD CALORIES: _____ / Daily Average: _____ Beginning Weight: _____

TOTAL ACTIVITY CALORIES: _____ Ending Weight: _____

Diet & Exercise Calendar

Name _____

Week Beginning _____

Daily Maintenance Calories _____ / Weekly _____

Daily Calories to lose 2 lbs/week _____ / Weekly _____

(Weekly = Daily x 7)

FOOD DIARY

Monday		Tuesday		Wednesday		Thursday		Friday		Saturday		Sunday	
Foods	Cal.	Foods	Cal.	Foods	Cal.	Foods	Cal.	Foods	Cal.	Foods	Cal.	Foods	Cal.
	Total:		Total:		Total:		Total:		Total:		Total:		Total:

EXERCISE DIARY

Minutes	Cal.	Minutes	Cal.	Minutes	Cal.	Minutes	Cal.	Minutes	Cal.	Minutes	Cal.	Minutes	Cal.
	Total:		Total:		Total:		Total:		Total:		Total:		Total:

Light Activity: 3 cal/min   Medium Activity: 5 cal/min   Heavy Activity: 7 cal/min

TOTAL FOOD CALORIES: _____ / Daily Average: _____

TOTAL ACTIVITY CALORIES: _____

Beginning Weight: _____

Ending Weight: _____

163

HWW HealthStyle Calendar

Daily Record of the Personal Goals Chart for the Month of _April_

Sunday	Monday	Tuesday	Wednesday	Thursday	Friday	Saturday
X=walked 1 mile calorie goal- less than 1500	(1250 calories) 1	(1500) X 2	(1100) 3	(1400) X 4	(1320) X 5	(1700) party 6
(900) 7	(1650) X 8	(1543) 9	(1200) X 10	(1253) 11	(1430) 12	(1425) X 13
(1189) 14	(1055) 15	(400) X 16	(1150) X 17	(1320) 18	(900) ↑ boss yelled at me! 19	(1421) 20
(853) 21	(1500) 22	(1150) 23	(1300) 24	(1253) 25 Business trip —	(1600) 26	(1900) 27
(1125) 28	(1293) X 29	(1326) X 30				

Record the progress of your personal goals, such as: total daily calories; days you exercise; days you abstain from a bad habit; days you complete a positive habit. Then, at the end of the month, transfer your results to your Personal Goals Chart.

HWW HealthStyle Calendar

Daily Record of the Personal Goals Chart for the Month of _____

Sunday	Monday	Tuesday	Wednesday	Thursday	Friday	Saturday

Record the progress of your personal goals, such as: total daily calories; days you exercise; days you abstain from a bad habit; days you complete a positive habit. Then, at the end of the month, transfer your results to your Personal Goals Chart.

MOTIVATION TIMELINE

Apply this motivation timeline to your Diet, Exercise & Mental Fitness Programs.

You should be adept at each stage before moving on. Time varies per person. Don't be concerned if a stage takes as long as a year. Remember, it is more than you were doing before.

STAGE 1 MOTIVATION: ESTABLISH THE HABIT

Weeks 1–7

1. Establish a routine. Nurture it. Take time to figure out the logistics of your new routine. Use rewards, progress charts, spouse support.
2. Be consistent. Adhere to your routine specifically. Give the momentum a chance to build.
3. Set lower-than-desired goals. Think "success" all the time.
4. Prioritize your program. Maintain a "no excuses" frame of mind, but . . .
5. No guilt. Learn to err gracefully.
6. Enjoy the process.

STAGE 2 MOTIVATION: BE YOUR OWN PSYCHOLOGIST

Weeks 8–15

1. Introduce *variety* to your routine if boredom is an issue (through new exercises or new recipes, for example).
2. Challenge yourself occasionally (extend your workout or leave half of your meal), but keep goals one notch lower than desired.
3. Analyze your excuses. Use Obstacle Chart that follows.
4. Be your own motivator. The new-program honeymoon has worn off by now and you'll need to pump yourself up occasionally.

STAGE 3 MOTIVATION: EVOLVE

Weeks 16–Forever

1. Experiment more with variety (some personality types require it more than others).
2. Goals can be more challenging, but be aware of overload.
3. Introduce flexibility. The advanced stage is less black and white—practice dealing with the "grays" of real life. Take

off a day if you need the rest (mental or physical). Experimentation and program alterations are in order, but make any changes *specific*. Eventually, you will learn to ebb and flow with your true needs and growth cycles.

4. Evolve. Think in terms of always refining your program (not necessarily tougher and tougher, but more fine-tuned to your specific needs). Hone your self-psychology and self-motivating skills. Learn, read, connect with others who have similar goals, know your vital statistics, and develop an interest in yourself.

NOT FUN
NOT
DONE

Chapter Nine

TAILORING YOUR WORKOUTS TO YOUR LIFE

THE HWW EXERCISE PROGRAM

You make taking care of your body a priority. One hour out of twenty-four isn't that much—my contribution to this corporation depends on my good physical shape.

— *Randy Barron, president, Southwestern Bell*

EXERCISE DOES EVERYTHING FOR YOU BUT MAKE YOU TALLER

I've always been aware of the machine of the body.
— Bruce Smart Jr., Continental Group

The findings on the health benefits of exercise are coming in so fast that it's hard for most people to keep up with them. For example, studies now link regular exercise with lower cancer rates—most recently with lower incidences of colon and breast cancer. Specifically, exercise causes your body to produce interluken and interferon, which strengthens your body's immune system, particularly against cancer. Given the chance, your body will take pretty good care of itself.

Your body is an amazing machine. You consist of 60 trillion cells, 600 muscles, 206 bones, and 60,000 miles of blood vessels. Your heart beats more than 100,000 times a day, and your kidneys filter 42 gallons of liquid a day. You make millions of new cells every minute, and your daily muscle work equals lifting 24 tons of material 4 feet high. As you can see, your body is truly a high-performance machine, and it should be carefully fueled and tuned so it can perform at its peak.

Researchers in the field of sports medicine are uncovering astounding information about the effects of exercise on aging. They've found that exercise actually helps slow the aging process. To be precise, exercise reverses reduced muscle tone and strength, limited flexibility, slowing reflexes, thinning bones, decreased lung capacity, decline of resting muscle oxygen intake, slowing metabolism, decline in ratio of muscle to fat, and weakening heart muscles. Exercise makes bone mass denser, preventing osteoporosis and brittleness that normally come with age. Furthermore, studies show that long-duration, low-intensity exercise such as walking significantly raises HDL levels (keeping the cholesterol ratio intact).

The symptoms of lack of exercise and aging are the same, and your biological age and chronological age can differ by as much as 25 years. A few years ago, the Mayo Clinic told my faithful-exerciser father that he had the body and health of someone twenty years younger. And, just like the soap commercials, my mother is often mistaken for my sister (she takes the *Walk*man literally). Don't think it's too late to begin, either. A study of men between 45 and 55 who had never exercised showed they could achieve levels of fitness almost equal to their peers who had exercised for ten or more years. Another study showed that seniors get even more out of exercise than do the young. Exercise increased the younger participants' functional capacity by 10 percent and the senior's by 50 percent. Makes you want to jump right on that Lifecycle, doesn't it?

Autopsies performed on more than 200 men and women who were 85 or older at death revealed that 30 percent had no dominant disease, and most of the remaining 70 percent had no disease that would be lethal during active middle age. Most died from the type of physical deterioration that exercise can prevent. Medical researchers are now saying that middle-aged exercisers can expect to live at least two to three years longer than their sedentary friends. Of course, some people argue that the promise of living longer is irrelevant, citing the "I-might-get-hit-by-a-truck-tomorrow" or "live for today" theories. However, they could hardly refute the benefits of having a higher *QUALITY* of life—right *NOW*. And that's the point: Exercise makes you feel and function better *today*, truck or no truck. Another plus for exercise—it improves sex lives. Studies show that people over 40 who exercise have sex lives like men and women in their late twenties. This may help explain the long marriages of these Captains of Industry.

COMPARE YOUR EXERCISE CHOICES WITH AMERICA'S MOST SUCCESSFUL

A comparison chart of exercises follows. It ranks and compares the favorite exercises of the HWW leaders with those of the American public in general. You can list your exercise preferences in the third column. Try not to look at or be influenced by the other columns until you have made your list.

Favorite Exercise List

HWW Leaders	American Public	Your Choices
#1 Running	#1 Walking	#1 _____
#2 Tennis/golf	#2 Swimming	#2 _____
#3 Bicycling	#3 Calisthenics	#3 _____
#4 Calisthenics	#4 Jogging	#4 _____
#5 Walking	#5 Bicycling	#5 _____
#6 Swimming	#6 Other active sports	#6 _____

If you had trouble coming up with a first choice (not to mention five more), you have plenty of company. More than four out of ten Americans are physically inactive. But why not change the course of your personal history right now? Use the blanks to list the forms of exercise you would now like to begin. Don't be too ambitious (hold off on mountain climbing for now), since this list is going to become your new exercise reality.

CAN THE FEET OUTRUN THE MOUTH?

Exercise reduces hunger. Specifically, *moderate* exercise reduces hunger—anything below 70 percent of maximum exertion turns glycogen into blood sugar that the body can use to fight the low blood sugar that makes you hungry. In addition, the hunger appestat in the brain (the hypothalamus) is affected by exercise and diminishes the desire to eat.

Exercise also counteracts the lowered metabolic rate (fat burning) incurred by reduced caloric intake. Even moderate exercise, such as half an hour of brisk walking a day, will do this. And, while you will lose solid fat if you include exercise with diet, you will lose both muscle and fat if you diet without exercise. Keep the muscle, since it helps you burn more calories and looks better than fat. Exercise along with dieting.

Exercise does allow some people to eat slightly more. Dow Chemical's CEO, Paul Oreffice, noticed that his weight problem disappeared when he returned to exercise after a long injury layoff. "I'm sorry, but now I can eat as much as I want," confesses Paul. (However, if you check his food intake in Chapter One you'll see that the foods Paul now enjoys aren't exactly calorie-laden. He also does not ingest extra hidden calories with cocktails—he only has about one drink a week.) Likewise, Southwestern Bell's president, Randy Barron, confesses, "I eat ice cream and I eat chocolate cake, but I can handle it if I exercise." In fact, if you've gone a little overboard on the ice cream or cake the night before, it's better for your health and energy level if you exercise 30 to 50 percent more the next day instead of starving yourself. (This is good to know as an occasional emergency measure, but be sure not to make this an ongoing self-punishing cycle.)

With all its merits, don't kid yourself about exercise and eating. Exercise alone won't take the weight off. Marathoner Emmett Smith of aerospace giant LTV, admits "I've struggled with diet all my life." Even when Smith ran over thirty-five miles a week, he still had to watch what he ate. "I have a hell of an appetite. I'll eat almost anything anyone puts in front of me." Emmett also has to watch his cholesterol level continually, and maintains, "Exercise is not a cure in and of itself." To lose one pound you'd have to run thirty-five miles or walk seventeen hours, take your pick. There is simply no way the feet can keep up with the mouth.

HOW MUCH EXERCISE DO YOU REALLY NEED?

Finding the ideal types and quantities of exercise for yourself is important for several reasons. First, exercise takes time, and time is valuable. Second, adherence requires a delicate psychological balance. And third, there is a point of diminishing returns in exercise, as well as an increased risk of injury. (You don't want to overdo it.)

If you want to exercise to lose weight, it is better to exercise longer and with a lower heart rate (60 percent of maximum versus 80 percent), because low-intensity, long-duration exercise (such as walking) burns more fat. High-intensity, short-duration exercise (such as aerobics or running) burns more carbohydrate calories than fat calories.

Exercising three to four times a week is said to be enough to maintain cardiovascular health, but it has been reported that you can lose weight three times faster if you exercise five times a week rather than three times a week.

Don't Punish Your Body.   Although most people don't need to be cautioned against overexercise, you should be aware that such a thing exists. Running more than 15 miles, doing more than four hours of aerobics, or doing any exercise more than twelve hours a week increases health risks and decreases benefits. In fact, athletes who burn more than 3,500 calories a week must take special care to supplement their diets and get extra rest so their bodies can repair themselves. Marathoners who speak of "hitting the wall" are talking about glycogen depletion, which can occur when strenuous exercise continues for more than two hours. When this happens, your body needs up to a week of recovery time to replace depleted muscle glycogen.

In our first conversation a few years ago, LTV's marathoner Emmett Smith spoke of the positive addiction aspect of exercise. He admitted he was hooked, running 100 miles a week for nine straight years. Then he came down with a bad flu that knocked him out of running for two weeks. When he started back in, he discovered that he was too much of a slave to his running program. Wisely, and with "a lot of willpower" he has removed rigidity from his program.

Unless you have the time and sincere interest to maintain a rigid workout schedule or complex training routine, don't torment yourself. Yes, it *is* necessary to make fitness a priority, but it is not necessary to dive into it with a cultlike mentality.

To help you get your exercise program going, here are a few motivating body-mathematic equations:

1. For each hour of physical activity, you can expect to live that hour over, and one or more to boot, according to Ralph Paffenbarger, M.D., University of Stanford.
2. The longer you exercise, the higher your artery-protecting HDL level becomes. Opt for distance over pace, says Terry Kavanagh, M.D., cardiologist at the Toronto Rehabilitation Center.

HEART RATE CALCULATIONS

Ideally, you should exercise at what is known as your Target Heart Rate for 30 to 40 minutes three to four times a week. There are several ways of calculating your Target Heart Rate. I consider the Karounen Method the best, since it takes your resting heart rate into consideration where other formulas do not. A person with a resting rate of 50 and a person of the same age who has a resting rate of 82 obviously should not have the same target heart rate range, even though they may be the same age. A pulse rate of 140 could be considered high for one person and low for the other.

Body Mathematics

Target Heart Rate: (Karounen Method)

220

− your age

− your one-minute resting pulse
(taken in the morning *before* you get out of bed)

× 0.60, .70, or .80 (beginner, intermediate, or advanced level)

+ your resting pulse

= Target Heart Rate

For example, you are 50 and have a resting heart rate of 70. You want to figure your medium-range intensity workout level, since you have been exercising regularly at an intermediate level.

220
− 50
− 70
× 0.70 (intermediate)
+ 70

140 = Target Heart Rate

Your Basic Fitness Equation Guide:

Duration: 30−40 minutes
Intensity: Target Heart Rate = 130−150 beats per minute
Frequency: 3−4 times per week

Recovery Heart Rate: The True Test

Along with monitoring your Target Heart Rate, you should check your Recovery Heart Rate when you are finished with your workout. Many consider this to be the true test in determining the health of your heart. After all, it's not just how fast and how long you get your heart beating but how quickly it comes back down to a normal pulse that's important. If your heart is still racing 20 minutes after exercising, you need to reassess your program.

How to Calculate Your Recovery Heart Rate

1. First, take your 1-minute pulse as soon as you've finished your workout. You can take a 6-second pulse and multiply by 10.
2. Wait one minute, then take your 1-minute pulse again.
3. Subtract this number from the first.
4. Now divide this number by 10.

Mathematically, the formula for determining your Recovery Heart Rate looks like this:

$$\frac{(\text{Exercise rate}) - (\text{One-minute-later rate})}{10} = \begin{array}{ll} 2 & (\text{poor}) \\ 3 & (\text{fair}) \\ 4{-}5 & (\text{good}) \\ 6{+} & (\text{excellent}) \end{array}$$

$$\text{Example:} \quad \frac{150 - 120 \,(= 30)}{10} = 3 \quad (\text{fair})$$

A person whose Recovery Heart Rate ranks "fair," as in the preceding example, should reduce exercise intensity (walk more slowly, for example). If your recovery rate is less than "good" (4 to 5), make your workouts a little easier for at least a week or so. Don't push it— you should be enjoying yourself!

THE KEY TO BEING CONSISTENT: "REGULAR RECURRENT" EXERCISE

Most of those in my study have a regular cardiovascular fitness routine that they do by themselves (requiring no partner), rain or shine, day in and day out. I call this Regular Recurrent Exercise, and it should be the foundation of your exercise program. Regular Recurrent Exercise is solitary, convenient, and excuse-free. It is one exercise or a combination of exercises that can be time-effective and at least palatable, if not somewhat enjoyable. If you don't enjoy repetition, however, this probably wouldn't be defined as "fun" (as in "Ha ha, I wish this would never end"). Regular Recurrent Exercise usually requires some commitment, at least until it becomes a habit.

There are two ways to approach Regular Recurrent Exercise:

1. Diversion Method (using diversions such as music, buddies, or note-taking to help take your mind off the fact that you are exercising).
2. Focus Method (using complete concentration on the exercise).

Many implement both methods in different circumstances, but you might do well to start with the Diversion Method. Both Robert McCowan of Ashland Oil and Bob Boni of Armco prefer using the Diversion Method. McCowan does his calisthenics and running in place at 6 A.M. while watching the news on TV. Music helped Boni get motivated with his exercise equipment after a knee injury in tennis. It was a definite adjustment for him, but the music made him stay with it, even after he was able to play tennis again. He now works out on a Lifecycle, rowing machine and treadmill while listening to jazz, big band and Dixieland music.

Athletes, on the other hand, usually stay with the Focus Method, having developed a positive response to the repetitive, meditative quality of this form of exercise.

The Benefits of Crosstraining.   Several forms of Regular Recurrent Exercises have been mentioned, including jogging, walking, calisthenics, bicycling, and the treadmill. It is a good idea to establish a rotating arsenal of Regular Recurrent Exercises, especially at the Stage 3 exercise level. This is known as *crosstraining*. While calisthenics or strength training are good, an aerobic workout should be your first priority in your Regular Recurrent itinerary

Strength Training.   The American College of Sports Medicine recently altered its fitness guidelines for the first time in twelve years to include a moderate amount of strength training. The recommendation is to include at least eight to ten resistance-type exercises involving the major muscle groups. Each exercise should be repeated eight to twelve times at a moderate intensity. This should be done at least twice a week and need not take more than fifteen minutes. You can use light weights to provide the resistance, or you can use your own body weight to provide the resistance and do the old standby calisthenics, such as leg lifts and pushups. These are Regular Recurrent Exercises that you can do virtually anywhere.

Because it is based on being solitary and convenient, Regular Recurrent Exercise helps simplify your exercise program and thus can ensure a higher adherence level. It also conditions you so that you can participate in sports more effectively and with fewer injuries. You should come up with one to four of your own favorite Regular Recurrent Exercises that you can—and will—do no matter what comes up, such as:

Rain.   Have indoor alternatives to outdoor exercises (for example, exercise videos, aerobic routines to your own favorite music, jumping rope, stationary bicycling, treadmill).

Injuries.   Be prepared. You'll be depressed, but don't let yourself make excuses. The alternative exercises you choose depend on the nature and extent of the injury, but bicycling and swimming are generally two good choices. If you can't move your lower body, exercise your upper body and vice versa.

Travel.   Same as Rain alternatives. And try to stay in hotels that have gyms, pools, or other exercise facilities.

Why You Should Get Hooked on a Sport

In addition to their Regular Recurrent daily conditioning, many of the men and women in my study have developed a sport interest that involves mastery and competition. When possible, sports should be encompassed into your HealthStyle program, because they add purpose and fun to your efforts.

Along with the camaraderie, you'll find many psychological advantages of sports that will carry over and enhance your job performance. Sports provide mental stimulation, playful competitiveness, interest and variety in life. Most important, it's yet one more reason to keep up their Regular Recurrent workouts. Running that extra half mile could just make the critical difference in that tennis match against "Iron Nerves Jamison" tomorrow, which makes it a challenge and keeps the exercise interesting.

Mixing Regular Recurrent Exercise and sports can create a balanced, self-motivating program. It is a formula that works for America's most successful. And it is a formula that can work for you.

THE THREE MOST IMPORTANT PARTS OF YOUR WORKOUT: WARMING UP, COOLING DOWN, AND STRETCHING

Warm Up.   Whether you simply want to stay in shape or are looking for some genuine physical challenges, you should begin any exercise routine slowly. Give your body at least five to seven minutes to warm up. Too many people start their early exercise efforts with a burst of enthusiasm and energy, only to have both wilt within minutes. Your heart needs time to catch up to the faster rate required of it, and your muscles need time to request (and get) more oxygen.

Cool Down.   After your workout, the first thing you need to do is to slow the heart rate down gradually from your aerobic range to a healthy recovery range. This should take 2 to 7 minutes, depending on the level of exercise intensity (refer to the Recovery Heart Rate formula on page 177). The cool down can be as simple as

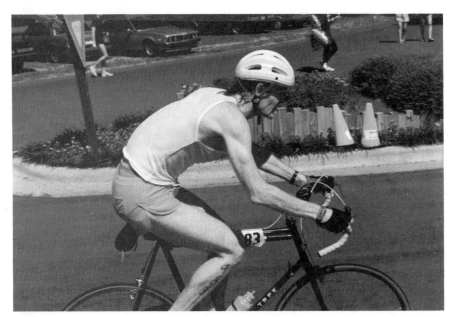

A triathlete with an impressively low cholesterol reading of 140, Brian Dyson of Coca-Cola Enterprises says his greatest personal achievement is maintaining a bodyfat ratio of 10.5 percent.

continuing your exercise activity in "slow-motion"; other times walking is a good cooldown choice.

Stretching.   The next thing you should do is stretch. Lactic acid levels will be as much as 50 percent lower if you stretch and cool down your muscles properly, preventing cramping, tearing, tightness, and soreness. One of the most impressive and surprising elements of the CEO workout is that so many incorporate stretches into their routines. Most of us know that stretching is a good thing, but figure we're lucky enough just to find the time to exercise, not to mention stretch. Besides, stretching really seems as if it should be reserved for serious athletes, right? Wrong. *Stretching is crucial for runners, walkers, bodybuilders and bicyclers at any level, and can significantly reduce your risk of injury.* If weight loss is the primary goal of your exercise, don't think of the warm up or cool down/stretch period as unproductive time—calories are still being burned.

While entire books have been written about stretching, let me simplify it for you. The point is to at least stretch the muscles that have just been used, because they have probably been shortened. The stretches hereafter described are pretty basic, but the trick is to do them correctly and hold them long enough or they will be ineffective at best and cause injury at worst. Treat each stretch like a yoga posture, that is, concentrate on the stretch instead of thinking of your marketing plan or gritting your teeth until it's over. You can thus simultaneously incorporate this time as your relaxation/meditation time.

Concentrating on the stretch means putting your focus on the muscle being stretched and then "breathing into it." Specifically, look at the tightest area with your mind's eye and allow it to relax; "see" the tension melting. Watch yourself sink deeper into the stretch with each exhalation. Relax, breathe, and let it go. You will notice minute releases with each exhalation, if you watch closely. Be careful not to try too hard and overstretch; this can cause injuries. Understretch, if anything. Always move slowly between stretches and *don't bounce during your stretch*. It is thought that we hold emotions (such as anger, frustration, or depression) in different parts of the body, so remember that it is not only exercise that can make muscles tight. The mind also plays a part. Conversely, the mind also can help a muscle relax. If stretches are performed with an open state of mind, you will probably feel some emotions release as the muscles release, giving you double benefit. In a brief, two- to seven-minute period, you can go to the clouds and back in terms of therapeutic relaxation— and stretch at the same time. If you need to shorten your overall workout time for some reason, shorten the exercise period rather than the stretch/cool down period, especially once you have reached the intermediate and advanced levels of exercising.

Initially, many people resist the stretching part of their program the most. Properly performed, however, the stretches can become a source of pleasure rather than an inconvenience. Put on some soft music. Give it a chance. Track stretches on your HWW HealthStyle Calendar on page 165 for just 30 days (with an X through each completed day) and you'll be on your way to a healthier, more toned and limber body. You may also notice a marked improvement in your posture as your muscles become more limber and balanced. Yogis believe that you are only as young as your spine is flexible.

FIVE POWER STRETCHES

1. Back/Hip/Leg/Arm/Chest/Neck

If you have time for only one stretch, this is the perfect choice. Lie on your back, legs together, arms stretched straight out from your shoulders, at a 90-degree angle from your body, palms down on the ground. Bend your right leg up so your foot is flat on floor, knee pointed toward ceiling. Roll toward the left, leaving your right shoulder on the ground. Hook your right foot behind your left straight leg, while you try to touch the floor with your right knee. Put your left hand on your right knee, guiding it downward while you look toward the right hand. Hold for at least 30 to 60 seconds. Then extend the lower right leg (calf and foot) to a straightened position with toe on the ground (right foot extending the same direction as left arm and parallel), heel toward ceiling. If you can reach, it is helpful to keep the left hand on the outstretched right leg for support. Keep looking at the right outstretched hand and breathe. Hold for at least 60 seconds. And now recite the Gettysburg Address.

2. Hamstring

This is the basic "touch your toes" hanging stretch. Your feet should be shoulder-width apart. Bend from the waist and let your arms and head hang down. Keep the knees "soft" (not locked). Touch the ground if you can, but don't force it. Breathe deeply, releasing the muscle tightness with each exhalation. Hold for at least 60 seconds.

3. Groin/Inner Thigh

Stand with your feet spread wider apart than your shoulders. Place the palms of your hands on the ground in front of you while bending your right knee into a lunge position, leaving your left leg straight. Feel the stretch on the left inner thigh. Hold for 30–60 seconds. Reverse. This stretch also gives the thigh muscles (quadriceps) a good workout.

4. Calf

The easiest method for calf stretching is to stand with the balls of your feet on the edge of a step or phone book so your heels hang over. Supporting yourself, bend your right knee while pushing down on the left heel. The left calf should be saying "yes" very quickly. Hold 30 to 60 seconds or longer while deep breathing and visualizing the muscle elongating. Repeat the procedure for the right calf.

5. Arm/Shoulder

In a standing or sitting position (this is a great exercise to do at your desk), clasp your hands behind your back with fingers in laced position. Straighten your arms and lift them up while arching the shoulders back without arching the lower back. This is an excellent tension reliever for the upper back and shoulders and is also wonderful for posture—it helps prevent stooping shoulders and concaving chest. Hold for 30 to 60 seconds. (Tip: turn your chair to the side, so you don't hit the back with your arms.)

TIPS:

For best results on all five stretches, remember to take your time and move slowly through the stretches, holding each one for at *least* 30 seconds. Concentrate on inhaling and exhaling during each stretch. If time is a problem, do one stretch properly rather than five that are rushed. Also, work stretching into your day, just as you do with exercise. Stretch while you are on the phone, in the elevator or even in the car.

THE HWW EXERCISE PROGRAM

How to Get Results: The Four Stages of the HWW Exercise Program

> People have a low chance of success if they are not in shape, and I hire accordingly.
>
> —Philip Smith, General Foods

The HWW Exercise Program is an evolutionary approach that will guide you from new exerciser to seasoned pro. The program includes four levels of exercise, each outlined hereafter. Important: To ensure success, start one level *lower* than where you think you should be. If you have not exercised in more than a month, start with Stage 1 Exercise Program—even if you are (or consider yourself) a "former athlete." The Stage 3 Exercise Program is really as far as you ever need to go. It provides the acceptable amount of exercise to maintain cardiovascular health. The Stage 4 Exercise Program, however, is for those who enjoy physical challenges, and it is the level pursued by many of the males I've discussed in this book.

The exercises listed in the four stages are arbitrary and are meant to be Regular Recurrent Exercises (ones that are convenient and that you can and *will* do alone). Make your choices based on your favorite forms of exercise you listed on the Favorite Exercise List, page 173. If you dislike walking, choose to swim or ride a bike. Walking is emphasized however, because it is an invaluable excuse-free Regular Recurrent "basic" to have in your repertoire. In the Stage 2 and Stage 3 programs, the sport interest is also arbitrary. But try to find a sport, even if it's one with fairly low activity, such as bowling. It will be better for you than sitting in front of the TV.

Notice that in Stage 1, you will start out exercising five times a week. The periods of exercise are short, of course, but the mind is being trained. As with all habits, *frequency* is emphasized over *intensity* or *duration* when you are trying to establish some consistency. If more than two days are missed at this critical stage, I have found that the delicate momentum is threatened. Some feel it is almost like starting over. You won't do any strength training at this stage—"one thing at a time . . ." In fact, you may want to wait a few months until you feel ready to add another aspect to your program. And if you have a real aversion to strength training (many people just can't stay with it for any length of time), don't worry. You will maintain a fit body without it. But try to incorporate some muscle-challenging activities into your day, such as stair climbing or carrying grocery bags to your car that you have purposely parked in the furthest space possible (see "No Time to Exercise" Program, page 186).

To calculate your particular intensity levels—low (beginning), medium (intermediate), high (advanced)—see Target Heart Rate (page 176). "Rest" days are optional—some prefer to keep the momentum going and exercise every day. Fine. Count the extra days as "Extra Credit." Stick to the schedule, however. It works.

General Tips:

1. Get a physical checkup before beginning this program. Also, make sure the doctor includes an HDL blood cholesterol test. Doctors often don't include this test in a physical unless it is requested.

2. Self-analyze and adjust as you go. Some days, weeks, or certain times of the year, you will be capable of doing more exercise—or less. These variations may be caused by a number of things, such as stress, sickness, biorhythms, or mood. The point is not to push yourself mercilessly through a regimented routine just because "this is what I am supposed to do on Thursdays." If you're feeling sluggish or fighting a minor virus, however, light exercise often can make you feel better (remember, exercise boosts the immune system). You may get started and find you can do more than you thought. The important thing is to do *something*.

STAGE 1 EXERCISE: CONVENIENT AND CONSISTENT

Weeks 1–7

1. Focus on convenience, simplicity.
2. Focus on *frequency* (over duration and intensity).
3. Calculate your Target Heart Rate *intensity* at 60 percent, low range, (page 176).
4. Monitor your Recovery Rate (see page 177).
5. Implement Stage 1 Motivation principles (see page 92).

What's happening at this stage is extremely important: you are establishing the habit of exercise! Exercise should be as pleasant and convenient as possible. You do not have to experience pain or even sweat—calories are still being burned! The main thing is to keep it up. You are teaching your body and mind to respond positively to a new thing. Most important, *you are establishing the habit of exercise.*

Stage 1 Exercise Schedule

Day	Warm Up (minutes)	Activity	Duration (minutes)	Intensity	Cool Down (minutes)
Monday	0	Walk	10–15	Low	2 (slow walk)
Tuesday	0	Walk	10–15	Low	2
Wednesday	0	Walk	10–15	Low	2
Thursday	Rest	Walk	10–15	Low	
Friday	0	Walk	10–15	Low	2
Saturday	0				2
Sunday	Rest				

Notice the simplicity (repetition of same exercise, walking). Your focus is on consistency rather than on avoiding boredom at this level. Boredom is not an issue yet, since the program is still new to you. In fact, I would encourage doing the same activity for these first few weeks to help get your pattern established. Psychologically, it is important at this level that you learn to handle the discrepancy between where you are and where you are going (a skill that will serve you in your career as well).

STAGE 2 EXERCISE: DURATION AND INTENSITY
Weeks 8–15

1. Increase exercise *duration*.

2. Increase *intensity* to 70 percent for at least two days a week, if ready.

3. Keep base program, but experiment with new activities if you feel the need.

4. Increase stretch time.

5. Implement Stage 2 Motivation principles (see page 93).

Stage 2 Exercise Schedule

Day	Warm Up (minutes)	Activity	Duration (minutes)	Intensity	Cool Down (minutes)
Monday	2	Walk	30	Low	2 (slow walk)
Tuesday	2	Walk	20–25	Medium	5
Wednesday	2	Bike*	10–15	Medium	5
		Strength**	5–10		
Thursday	Rest				
Friday	2	Walk	30	Low	2
Saturday	2	Bike	10–15	Medium	5
		Strength	5–10	Low	
Sunday	Rest				

*"Bike" can be a stationary bike or other aerobic equipment such as rowing machine, stair machine, treadmill, and so forth. (Check newspaper want ads for good second-hand equipment.)
**"Strength" means Strength Training.

STAGE 3 EXERCISE: INCREASE DURATION, INTENSITY, ADD VARIETY

Weeks 16–23 (or forever)

1. Increase *intensity* up to 80 percent at least 2 days a week.
2. Increase *duration*.
3. Add variety.
4. Increase Stretch time.
5. Implement Stage 3 Motivation principles (see page 93).

STAGE 4 EXERCISE: CROSSTRAIN

Weeks 23–Forever

1. Crosstrain to avoid injuries and boredom.
2. Increase *duration, frequency, intensity*.
3. Increase stretch time.
4. Extend walks (45 to 60 minutes) at 60 to 65 percent intensity for more fat burning.
5. Implement Stage 4 Motivation principles (see page 94).

THE "NO TIME TO EXERCISE" PROGRAM

Sometimes you may think you have no time at all for an exercise program, *but you do*—and remember that every little bit helps. Here are some simple tips for snatching fitness moments at work or at home.

Stage 3 Exercise Schedule

Day	Warm Up (minutes)	Activity	Duration (minutes)	Intensity	Cool Down (minutes)
Monday	2	Walk	30–45	Low	2 (slow walk)
Tuesday	5	Bike*	20	High	5–7
		Strength**	15	Medium	
Wednesday	3	Walk	30–40	Medium	3–5
Thursday	Rest (or golf, etc.)				
Friday	5	Bike	20	High	5–7
		Strength	15		
Saturday	2	Walk	30–45	Low	2 (slow walk)
Sunday	Rest (or golf, etc.)				

*The two low-intensity days can be exchanged for shorter duration, higher intensity (medium) days, if desired.
**"Strength" means Strength Training (see page xxx).

Stage 4 Exercise Schedule

Day	Warm Up (minutes)	Activity	Duration (minutes)	Intensity	Cool Down (minutes)
Monday	2	Walk	45–60	Low	2
Tuesday	5–7	Tennis	60–90	Med–High	5–7
		Strength**	15–30	Med–High	
Wednesday	Rest (or golf, etc.)				
Thursday	5–7	Bike	30	High	5–7
		Strength	15–30	Med–High	
Friday	5–7	Walk/Jog	30–40	Med–High	5–7
Saturday	5–7	Bike	30	High	5–7
		Strength	15–30	Med–High	
Sunday	2 (or golf, etc.)	Walk	45–60	Low	5

**"Strength" means Strength Training (see page xxx).

1. Desktop Pushups

Getting down on the floor to do pushups is often inconvenient and just awkward enough to discourage the intention altogether. So, for a quick 10-second to 60-second upper body workout, almost any time, any place, try desktop pushups. Stand about 3 to 4 feet away from a desk or counter top. Place the palms of your hands on the edge of the desk or counter top. Make a straight angle of your body from the back of your head to the back of your heels. Now, keeping your body straight, bend your elbows until your chin almost touches the desktop or counter top while lowering your body. Then straighten your elbows and lift your body back up. Do as many desktop pushups as you can—you will quickly build up strength and muscles. Do them at your desk between calls for a quick energizer or at your sink before going to work in the morning or going to bed. Do a set of 10, then brush your teeth, do another set, then wash your face, do another set, then get dressed. This exercise will shape the entire upper body: chest, back, shoulders, upper arms, and midriff area.

2. TV Fat Burner

Commit to getting up and moving around (exercise or just getting things done) during every television commercial three nights a week. However, start with one show, one night. This presents a good opportunity to get a lot of little things done and keeps your metabolism up (just the act of standing up increases your heart beat 10 beats per minute).

3. Power Shopping or Briefcase Weights

Walk to the grocery store instead of driving. Request the handle-type plastic bags and divide the groceries' weight evenly between the two bags. Walk home carrying your "bag weights" in each hand. As you walk, lift and lower the bags by bending your elbows (one at a time or together). Rest for a block when your arms get tired and then do another "rep" (repeat the arm exercise). I watched one executive build up his upper body and lose 25 pounds in six months doing nothing but this and eating slightly smaller portions—at an earlier hour. (He shopped and walked six to seven nights a week.) This exercise can also be done with your briefcase.

4. Clean-Up Workout

Do housework, laundry, and car washing yourself. You can get a great two-hour workout every Saturday morning by doing the laundry and housecleaning simultaneously. Put on your headset and let the party begin! If nothing else, go for a walk during the wash or dry cycles. Don't sit and wait.

5. Walking Meetings

Double up social or business appointments with exercise time. Walk with your associates instead of sitting in a stuffy office filled with interruptions. "Talking walks" promote creative conversational flow.

Also, redefine your entertainment and relaxation time with spouse and friends. Make this time active: an adventurous hike, a game of tennis, or rowing a boat on a lake. Don't think of it as exercise. Just enjoy the camaraderie and watch the relationship expand.

6. Tight Spot Exercises: Isometrics

Do isometric exercises at your desk, in conferences, on planes, or in the car. Tighten and release the muscles in your stomach, buttocks, thighs, biceps, one area at a time. Tighten for the count of 10. Release. Repeat until muscle is exhausted. Then go to next area. When finished with all areas, start over and do another complete round or two. This can also be done with a faster rhythm: one second for each muscle contraction and one second for each release. Keep time to your favorite upbeat music (in your car for example) by contracting and releasing with the beat. Repeat for 25–50–100 beats (until muscle is exhausted).

7. Walk Stairs

You've heard it before. Here it is again: Don't take the elevator. People are now paying big bucks for stair machines. But any flight of stairs will give you the same exercise—free! Just think of that back stairwell as your own very elite exercise equipment . . .

Every Little Bit Helps

Physical exertion translates to calories being burned, which translates to pounds being lost. The following should help impress the "every little bit helps" philosophy.

Exercise:	Yearly Loss (calories expended)
1. 30-minute walk (7 times a week)	18 lbs
2. Car or desk isometrics (5 times a week, 10 minutes)	4 lbs
3. Wash car (1 time a week, 30 minutes)	2.3 lbs
4. Walk during TV commercials (for 12 viewing hours per week)	2 lbs
5. Stair climbing (7 times a week, 2 flights, up and down)	6 lbs
TOTAL POUNDS:	32.3 lbs (That's a small person!)

TIPS
TO REMEMBER:

- *Exercise 30 to 50 percent more instead of starving yourself after overeating.*
- *It's never too late to begin—seniors can get even more out of exercise than do the young.*
- *Exercise helps slow the aging process.*

MIND
OVER
MOUTH

Chapter Ten

EATING FOR BODY, MIND, AND CAREER POWER

THE HWW DIET & NUTRITION PROGRAM

Some people let their bodies go to pot. They don't balance their lives—it's always a crash program.

—Dr. Bob Boni, Armco

For best results, you should view the HWW Program as much as an internal process as an external one; as much about your thinking process as about what goes on your plate. This chapter will give you both—some food for thought as well as suggestions on food to eat. *What* you eat, how *much* you eat and how *often* you eat can have a strong effect on your exercise program, on your ability to think clearly at crucial times and, ultimately, on achieving your goals.

One of the first things you must consider before launching into a HealthStyle improvement program is your personality. Are you a perfectionist/non-perfectionist; introvert/extrovert; optimist/pessimist; Type A/Type B? We all think we know ourselves pretty well, but it is worth a minute or two of your time to think this one through and then gear your program accordingly. If you don't, you may put a lot of energy into the wrong approach and fail. I have structured the HWW Diet & Nutrition Program to allow you the freedom to customize your approach; to consider your individual likes, dislikes, needs, and goals. For example, while I suggest counting

195

calories as a good way to know exactly how much you are ingesting in the beginning learning stage, there are other methods. If you rebel at the idea of counting calories, you can limit quantity in other specific ways and get the same results (see Evolutionary Approach, page 216). The idea is not to kid yourself about your food intake.

The HWW Diet & Nutrition Program lays out a specific schedule that makes weight loss painless and even enjoyable. The idea, however, is to start trusting your new health-educated self more and relying less on outside sources with quick, generic answers and "magic" diets. Believe it or not, you are the one most capable of knowing the needs of your body.

QUICK COMPARISON TEST: HOW YOUR DIET STACKS UP

It can be interesting and enlightening to compare your favorite foods with those of America's most successful. The following "test" will give you a pretty good feel of where you stand in comparison. You may be pleasantly surprised or a little disappointed. But don't feel bad if you are not yet having the breakfast, lunch, or dinner of champions. I intend for this comparison to serve as a motivational "shocker" for any donut-loving champions-to-be who need one last shot of motivation before starting the program.

To participate in the test, quickly list your four all-time favorite foods, without looking at the HWW list below. Be honest. Now compare your list with the all-time favorite of the HWW leaders. (Yes, they were specifically asked to consider everything from chocolate cake to T-bone steaks.)

Favorite Food List

HWW Leaders' All-Time Favorite Foods:	Your All-Time Favorite Foods:
#1 Fish	#1 _____
#2 Salad	#2 _____
#3 Fruit	#3 _____
#4 Chicken	#4 _____

If your list doesn't look much like the executive list, you might want to use some of the psychological techniques described in Chapter Five to start changing your tastes. While fish may never make your favorite-food list, you could certainly begin keeping a good supply of fresh fruits around to eventually replace those potato chips.

THE FEEDING OF A CHAMPION

Following is a list of the foods most commonly eaten by some of America's most successful people. It ranks the frequency with which each item was eaten. Note that some items often were combined. If you modify your eating choices to match these items, you will be in good dietary shape.

BREAKFAST CHOICES: (6–7 A.M.)

   #1 Cereal (whole grain, no sugar cereal with nonfat milk)

   #2 Toast (whole wheat, often dry)

   #3 Eggs (poached)

   #4 Fruit

   #5 Bran muffin

   #6 Pancakes (weekend treat)

   #7 Yogurt

LUNCH CHOICES: (11:30 A.M.–12:30 P.M.)

   #1 Salad (tuna or chicken)

   #2 Soup (clear or vegetable)

   #3 Sandwich (tuna or turkey, no mayonnaise)

   #4 Fish (broiled swordfish is popular)

   #5 Vegetable

   #6 Chicken

   #7 Red meat

       No dessert!

DINNER CHOICES: (6–7 P.M.)

   #1 Vegetables

   #2 Fish

   #3 Chicken

   #4 Red meat

   #5 Varied entree (pasta is popular)

   #6 Fruit

       No dessert!

Following are some meal recommendations based on the food preferences of the leaders in my study, as well as other information.

You can choose the meals that best suit your needs and taste buds and rotate them for variety, or apply the suggestions and create your own meals, using similar nutrition and caloric guidelines (depending on your weight loss goals).

Amounts are calculated to be a typical serving, but measure your own amounts exactly and check calories at first, especially if calorie-counting is new to you. Regardless of calories, however, remember to eat only until you are *satisfied* rather than *full*. Change the diet-as-jail mentality to the *choice* mentality and use the new techniques you've learned in this book. Meals are based on the recipes given in Chapter 11. (Chapter 12 offers a comprehensive menu plan and teaches you how to shop, cook, and coordinate menus by the day, week, and month.)

Breakfasts of Champions

1. Whole grain, no sugar cereal or oatmeal, nonfat milk
   Juice or strawberries or blueberries
   Decaffeinated coffee or herb tea
   TOTAL CALORIES   200

2. Bran muffin
   Banana   TOTAL CALORIES   340

3. Toast (two pieces, whole wheat)
   English muffin or bagel
   Fruit
   Yogurt   TOTAL CALORIES   370

Breakfast Tips: See "Eight Great Breakfast Ideas," Chapter 12, for more ideas.

MILK

Try to get accustomed to nonfat milk or Yogurt Milk (see Recipes). If either seems too watery at first, try adding some powdered milk. This will add flavor, nutrition, very few calories, and no fat. If you anticipate resistance from family members, don't tell them at first. Use whole milk cartons and make the change like a thief in the night.

FRUIT

Opt for whole fruit instead of juice, if possible. You get more for your money: more nutrition, fiber, bulk, and taste, but fewer calories. Also, you won't get such a sudden rise and fall of blood sugar (energy level) with whole fruit as you will with juice. The sugars in juice are natural, but don't let that fool you. They will boost your energy for an hour or so, then your blood sugar level will drop, leaving you with the morning blahs just when you need to be the most alert. This is particularly true if juice is consumed alone or if you have hypoglycemia (low blood sugar). If you insist on having juice, try making a spritzer with half juice and half sparkling water. Incidentally, it is wise to eat fruit first at a meal, so it will be able to move more quickly through your system.

COFFEE VERSUS HERBAL TEAS

Drink decaffeinated if you must drink coffee, but think about gradually substituting herbal teas as you evolve your diet. Even decaf is considered a dietary "minus" (it has some caffeine, and some brands are made with a process that is considered carcinogenic). On the other hand, most herbal teas can actually be a "plus" (camomile has a calming effect and rose hip tea can give you a vitamin C boost).

TOAST

Invest in good bread. This means using the most nutritious, best-tasting bread you can find. You may have to visit a health-food store across town once a month, but it is worth it. If you can't get to a health-food store, check the ingredients of the breads sold at the supermarket. Look for breads with whole wheat flour and very few other things. You don't want sugar, preservatives, or ingredients you can't pronounce. With breads, do *not* shop price or calories; shop taste. Half a piece of hearty bread is more satisfying than a whole loaf of tasteless low-calorie bread. If you keep your bread frozen and take it out as needed, it will be fresh and nutritious for you daily. Put it right from the freezer into the toaster. If you want to make a sandwich, remove it from the toaster after about one minute (before it becomes toast).

If you are looking for a creative dietary outlet, consider making your own bread, as Malcolm Stamper of Boeing does. Homemade bread can give you optimum nutrition, great taste, and a sense of accomplishment as well. For additional flavor, try all-fruit, no-sugar or low-sugar spreads.

MUFFINS

As with breads, invest in good muffins. For best results, you can make your own (see Multiway Muffins in Chapter 11) or get someone to make them for you. The advantage with homemade muffins is that you can customize your own and cut down on calories by eliminating the oil. Also, you can opt to use rice or oat flour and bran in your muffin if you have high cholesterol or wheat allergy problems. Or you can make them with wheat bran if you have a problem with constipation. Use a combination of both brans if you want both benefits. You also can add raisins, nuts, apples, shredded carrots (great for lowering cholesterol), and other items. Make or buy nutritious muffins in large quantities and freeze them. Heat one up while you take your morning shower.

YOGURT

Buy plain yogurt that has 100 to 160 calories per cup. Choose the large, 32-ounce size and custom flavor the entire container at one time. Add fructose or dry barleymalt sweetener (Dr. Bronner's) with a dash of flavoring, such as vanilla or strawberry and/or fresh fruit pieces. An added tip: fill champagne glasses with yogurt, put a strawberry (or other piece of fruit) on top, sprinkle with bran, and freeze. Remove from freezer as you begin your meal and it will partially thaw into a delicious 50-calorie dessert.

Lunches of Champions

1. Broiled swordfish
   Steamed vegetables (broccoli, carrots)
   Baked potato   TOTAL CALORIES   325
2. Tuna salad
   Fruit   TOTAL CALORIES   350
3. Turkey sandwich (no mayonnaise)
   Vegetable soup   TOTAL CALORIES   475

Lunch Tip: Eat fruit first or save for between-meal snack.

Brown Bag Suggestions:

1. Tuna sandwich (made with HWW "Mayo"—see Chapter 11)
   Rice chips (by Amsnack or Rice Bites by American Grains)
   Apple
2. Turkey or chicken sandwich
3. Pasta salad (with HWW salad dressing—see Chapter 11)
4. Yogurt (sweetened with natural sweetener and sprinkled with raw granola)
   Fruit
5. Soup—homemade (if access to microwave)
   Whole-wheat crackers or muffin
   Salad—tuna, turkey, cottage cheese (if refrigerator at work)
7. Vege-Sandwich (with grated carrots, tomatoes, sprouts/lettuce, avocado, cucumber, HWW "Mayo," Dijon mustard, and so forth)

8. Last night's healthy leftovers (Chapter 11 recipes)—cold or heated in the microwave.

Dinners of Champions

1. Steamed vegetables over rice
   Whole wheat roll
   One glass of wine   TOTAL CALORIES   450
2. Poached salmon
   Carrot salad
   Baby red potatoes   TOTAL CALORIES   375
3. Chicken
   Vegetable salad
   1 glass wine   TOTAL CALORIES   550

Snacks of Champions

Morning:

1. Fresh fruit   CALORIES   60–70

Afternoon:

1. Unsalted raw almonds (5–10)
2. Fruit
3. Yogurt (¾ cup, barleymalt-sweetened, nonfat, plain)
                                        CALORIES (each) 70–100

Evening:

1. Crudites (with yogurt dip, optional)
2. Popcorn (no butter)
3. Fruit   CALORIES (each) 100

SAMPLE HWW POWER DIET

If you think you have grasped the HWW diet concept and are eager to get started, that's great—skip to the HWW Diet & Nutrition Program later in this chapter. However, if you feel as if you need a bit more structure, a sample weekly menu to get you going is presented here. Remember that, ultimately, it's up to you to make good eating habits an enjoyable part of your life. This takes an initial investment of time to learn what eating right is all about and how to incorporate the proper foods into your life. Be persistent. Exper-

A HWW Power Menu

Day	Breakfast	Lunch	Dinner
Monday	oatmeal strawberries juice	tuna salad apple	chicken carrot salad roll
Tuesday	wheat toast banana yogurt	vegetable soup carrot salad fruit juice-sweetened cookie	salmon steamed vegetables rice pilaf
Wednesday	whole-grain cereal banana	turkey sandwich peach	pasta salad salad
Thursday	whole-grain cereal blueberries	broiled snapper salad	lean steak vegetable roll
Friday	oatmeal peach	tostada	swordfish baked potato salad
Saturday	whole-grain cereal banana	cold chicken fruit plate fruit juice-sweetened cookie	pizza salad
Sunday	pancakes grapefruit	vegetable soup salad	Chinese food frozen yogurt
Snacks	fruit; cold, skinned chicken; raw vegetables; popcorn without butter		

202

iment. Find the foods you like. If what you really want is cabbage and carrots for breakfast, such as J. C. Penney's David Miller, or oatmeal and blueberries for dinner, do your thing.

The men and women I studied truly *enjoy* life—including the food they eat to sustain it. "We enjoy a robust life," says Malcolm Stamper, "and our food complements it. We like what we eat." Stamper loves to cook and over the years he has completely changed his eating habits from those of his childhood. He claims he has even lost his taste for butter and salt.

The sample HWW Power Menu more clearly illustrates how America's most powerful executives dine, day in and day out. This diet is a good place to start if you'd like a specific weekly guide to get you rolling. The meals are simple but tasty and nutritious, and they require no complicated recipes, ingredients, or cooking techniques. They use whole foods, which are better for you (more vitamins and bulk). You can adapt this menu easily to your lifestyle, whether you travel, eat in restaurants, are single, or cook for your family.

FIVE DIET DON'TS

If you are trying to lose weight, first let's talk about how not to diet:

1. Don't eat foods to which you are allergic. How do you know if you are allergic? Foods that you can't stop eating are often allergy foods. Other symptoms of food allergy are wide-ranging, including hives, weight gain, headaches, stomach distress and bloating, and throat mucus. Tune in to subtle or blatant symptoms and consider those foods you have recently ingested. Be your own detective. No weight-loss program stands a chance against food allergies.

2. Don't go on a crash calorie diet. In 1990, 20 million Americans spent nearly $1 billion on liquid diets (many were medically supervised—meaning doctors are condoning them!). The facts are coming in too hard and fast to ignore now: *The safest way to lose weight is with a balanced deficit diet (well-balanced, but moderately lower in calories).* The body can only lose two or three pounds of fat a week—the rest is water. If you cut your caloric intake too drastically, the body goes into a starvation protection mode. It produces and releases Reverse T3, an adaptive hormone that counters the perceived threat of starvation by lowering body metabolic rate. In this "starvation state," your body adapts to 25–40 percent fewer calories than normal. The consequence is that you will gain weight on the same amount of calories on which another person would be losing weight. Wouldn't you rather eat those calories and lose weight anyway? Crash dieting can permanently alter your metabolism, making it harder than ever to lose weight for the rest of your life. This may be one reason why women have more difficulty losing than men (since they tend to diet more). Another reason is that women's body fat ratio is higher than men's. Interestingly, very few in my study have ever tried the starvation method or any other fanatical approach to weight loss.

3. Don't go on a food-group elimination diet.   Rice or grapefruit diets, protein-only diets, and other food-group elimination schemes can throw your body chemistry way off balance, causing stress to your digestive and immune systems and robbing you of nutrients in the process. Such diets also can affect your "braincomputer." Foods are simply chemicals that produce various neurotransmitters (brain messengers). Feed the brain an imbalance of nutrients, and an imbalance is what will be transmitted. Specifically, erroneous messages will be translated. For example, sugar often triggers the message, "I'm hungry, keep eating" (since sugar is essentially a nonfood, and the body is craving something nutritiously satisfying). A better message in this case would be, "Enough junk food. Now feed me something nutritionally satisfying." USA Network's Kay Koplovitz once tried an apple-only diet in support of a dieting friend. She had to quit after she developed migraine headaches. (Kay says she no longer "actively" supports dieting friends.) Cut calories and fat, not food groups.

4. Don't go on a prescribed daily menu diet.   Don't follow daily menus or lists of foods you can or can't eat. We're talking lifetime here, and you don't want to face grapefruit and one slice of dry toast every Wednesday morning for the rest of your life whether you like it or not. You're much better off weaning yourself from unhealthful foods, culling the most healthful of the foods you already like, and adding to your repertoire over time through a little fun and creativity in the kitchen.

5. Don't chew gum.   Gum stimulates the salivary glands (which makes you hungry) and tightens the jaw muscles (which can aggravate stress and cause headaches).

SIX CRITICAL EATING TRAPS TO AVOID

At least six common circumstances can contribute to "miseating" (clinical terminology for pigging out). You can add your own circumstances to this list and try to come up with some solutions for them, as I have done. (Refer to "How to Troubleshoot HealthStyle Obstacles," page 100.) Then, when they pop up, you will have already outsmarted them, both psychologically and logistically and will thus have eliminated one more deterrent to staying on your HealthStyle path.

Eating Trap #1: **Eating over Emotions, Tiredness, or Thirst**

Tiredness, depression and thirst are not hunger (a good motivational sign to post on your refrigerator). Whenever you feel the urge to eat beyond your limit, analyze your motives. Ask yourself if you are really tired (try to catch a cat nap or take a few deep breaths), depressed (sit it out, meditate, or talk to a friend), or thirsty (drink some water). Wait five minutes. Realize that an excuse to eat is trying to manifest. Be willing to experience hunger and remember: Hunger means fat is burning.

Bruce Smart says that when he is short on sleep, he notices the desire to eat more (eating raises blood sugar and energy levels—temporarily). Armco's Dr. Bob Boni says, "I have a theory that diet and stress interrelate. Stress can exacerbate the situation" (cause you to eat more). If you pay close attention to the reasons you overeat, however, you will not only lose weight, but will also lose the deep-rooted causes that led to overeating (or any other self-destructive or compulsive behavior) in the first place. Weight loss then becomes a well-deserved bonus to self-development.

Eating Trap #2: **Skipping Meals While on the Run**

Be prepared. It is not macho or "big business" to skip meals. This can contribute to dull thinking, low energy, ulcers, and gaining weight. Keep a stash of emergency foods on hand for those unpredictable times when normal meal times are postponed or missed. Stock your briefcase, purse, desk, or glove compartment with allowable, healthful snacks, such as fruit or muffins. (This does not include sweets, potato chips, and other recreational edibles.)

Eating Trap #3: **"Anything Goes on Weekends" Mentality**

Develop a Weekend Spa Mentality. Many of the men and women I spoke with look forward to the weekends as a time to really get into gear with their HealthStyle efforts. They avoid the "Anything goes on the weekends" mentality. Remind yourself that you deserve to arrive at work Monday morning energized and cleansed, not hung over from two days of over-indulgence. Resolve to savor special meals during the weekend and forgo snacks entirely or vice versa.

Eating Trap #4: **Overeating at Restaurants**

If you are planning to eat out and are exceptionally hungry, eat a *little* healthful snack before leaving your house or order a lo-cal appetizer (shrimp cocktail) as soon as you arrive to avoid devouring quantities you'll later regret. Colombe Nicholas, president emeritus of Christian Dior, says, "When you're an executive and dine out a great deal and entertain a lot, it's so easy to eat too much." Her secrets? "I order things like artichokes that take forever to eat and keep my hands busy." If she must wait for someone and she is hungry, she will drink a large glass of water or tell the waiter to bring a small salad immediately. Her tip for eating buffet style is to "Look at the whole thing and decide what you really want. If it's cake, have it and skip the rest—not on a regular basis, of course. But you must break the tradition of having to have the entire course."

Order dressings and sauces on the side or not at all. Order fish, vegetables, baked potatoes. Best of all, try not to eat out so much. Paul Oreffice reports, "I eat out as little as possible. My treat is to eat at home. I'm in charge of the salad dressing."

Eating Trap #5: **Overeating on Vacations and Business Trips**

Eating on the road is tough for the execs, although several, including Kathryn Klinger, beat the added difficulty by simply using road time as dieting time. Columbe Nicholas' road rules include drinking a lot of water and avoiding alcohol. Never use travel as an excuse to overeat. Of the execs in my study who rated tops in diet, over half travel more than ten weeks a year—proof that eating correctly on the road can be done.

To avoid becoming a Wide Load while on the road, track your food intake and exercise more, if necessary, to avoid nibbling and overindulging. However, don't try to be a perfectionist about eating exactly the way you do at home. This will lead to frustration and more overeating. Learn how to improvise gracefully.

Eating Trap #6: **The Bachelor(ette) Mentality**

You don't always have to eat out. You can learn the basics of cooking and do an excellent job of taking care of yourself. Have a health-oriented friend or mother show you how to boil water, steam vegetables, bake potatoes, poach fish, and do other healthful basics. This is a worthwhile project, since dining out on a continuous basis will put weight on your body and take weight off your bank account. For the same cost as eating out (or less), you can hire someone to stock your refrigerator once a week with the basics, as described in The Speed Cooking Plan (such as a big salad, soup, fruit, good whole-wheat rolls and bread, chicken). With very little effort, you can eat the most healthful, tasty meals in your own home. The kitchen no longer has to be considered foreign territory. If you must indulge in frozen foods from the grocery store, check labels carefully for sodium and fat content.

HOW MUCH CAN YOU EAT AND STILL LOSE WEIGHT?

To stay healthy and live longer, one of the most important things you can do is to eat less, contends one of America's foremost authorities on both gerontology and the benefits of undereating. UCLA gerontologist Roy Walford, M.D., believes that we can decrease by half the rate at which we age; that we can live to be 120 by intelligent (nutritious) undereating. Overeating severely taxes the body, much like an alcoholic binge. Among other things, men who are 30 percent overweight have a 70 percent higher risk of heart disease. Overweight women have higher risks of contracting cancer. In contrast, people who weigh 10 percent less than average for their height tend to have significantly longer lifespans.

As you get older, you should reduce the quantity of what you eat while increasing the quality. With every decade, your need for calories lessens by 2 percent, while your need for certain vitamins and minerals—such as calcium, for example—increases. If you keep your eating habits the same from year to year, you will gain an average of two pounds a year, or twenty pounds a decade.

Remember that "leave something on your plate" advice that came with every diet you have ever tried? Your internal response probably was something like mine: "Yeah, right. Leave a precious morsel behind—one that I am legally entitled to—and do it for no apparent reason? Fat chance." ("Fat" is not used inadvertently here. It is generally what happens when you eat every last one of your treasured bites.) Actually, leaving a small amount of food is a good first step in developing food-stomach-mind awareness. This act opens a huge door to becoming your own teacher, tuning in to your true needs, and breaking old, mechanical eating habits. A naturally thin friend of mine made dinner for me one evening, preparing my plate with an arbitrary portion of food. After I had "licked my platter clean," he asked if I would like more. I declined in a very ladylike manner. Teasing, he said, "Come on. That had to be either too much or too little. It couldn't have been just the exact right amount to the bite. I don't understand why people eat exactly what was on their plates." I thought about it later and realized that he was quite right and that this was, in fact, a rather useful insight. I started giving just a bit more consideration as to when the end of my meal should officially take place (with his laughing image sitting on my shoulder). Soon, it became second-nature to stop when my body signaled, instead of when the signal came from my eyes, emotions or habits. Start experimenting by leaving something on your plate each time you dine and watch how that opens up a whole new concept in eating.

EVERY LITTLE BIT ADDS UP: TEN DIETARY PAYOFFS

Now that you are becoming calorie-aware, the following chart will help you see how those calories add up—and add pounds. You can also see how easy it is to make a few simple HealthStyle changes that permit the weight to come off on its own.

Ten Dietary Payoffs

	Yearly Loss (calories saved)
Exchanges	
1. Baked potato instead of French fries (3 times a week, 4 oz. each)	10 lbs.
2. Vegetable soup vs. creamed soup or chili (3 times a week)	7.8 lbs.
3. Broiled chicken vs. fried chicken (2 times a week, 6 oz.)	4.5 lbs.
4. Nonfat milk vs. whole milk	7.3 lbs.
Yogurt milk (see Speed Cooking Plan) vs. nonfat milk	*6.8 lbs.
Yogurt milk vs. whole milk *(7 times a week, 8 oz.)	*14 lbs.
5. Lo-cal salad dressing vs. regular (2 tablespoons a day)	12.5 lbs.
6. Fish (broiled) vs. sirloin steak (broiled) (2 times a week, 4 oz.)	7.9 lbs.
7. Turkey sandwich (no mayo) vs. hamburger ("the works")	8.9 lbs.
Eliminations	
8. Mayonnaise (1 tablespoon a day)	10.5 lbs.
9. Dessert (5 days a week)	22 lbs.
10. Alcoholic beverages (5 days a week, 2 drinks per night)	14.8 lbs.
TOTAL POUNDS SAVED:	105.6–113 lbs.
	(That's a whole person!)

A FAILPROOF FORMULA FOR LOSING WEIGHT

Calories. We've come full circle in the weight-loss battle, and there's no escaping it: To lose weight, you must establish the proper balance between caloric intake and caloric expenditure (physical activity). It's basic math. Remember, the consensus among weight loss experts now is that *the safest way to lose weight is with a balanced deficit (in calories) diet.*

To lose one to three pounds a week, the general consensus among dietary experts is that women should eat no more than 1,000 to 1,200 calories a day, and men should limit their calories to about 2,000 a day. See the following formula to determine your exact daily caloric allowance. Keep track for 60 to 90 days using your HWW Diet & Exercise or HealthStyle Calendar. You will soon learn to "eyeball" amounts. For example, a portion of rice the size of a deck of cards is 135 calories (6 oz.), and a bit of butter the size of a quarter (½ teaspoon) is 25 calories.

The popular concept now is that you *get* fat by *eating* fat. True. But you also get fat by eating too many calories—of *any* kind! Thus, counting calories should be the primary focus in your Stage 1 Eating Program. More attention will be placed on what *kinds* of calories you are consuming in Stage 2. This is important because, indeed, *all calories are not created equal.* A fat calorie has a greater potential for increasing body fat than a carbohydrate calorie does. In other words, 50 calories worth of carrots is not the same as 50 cookie calories.

Here is another calorie fact to incorporate into your diet: *When* you eat is almost as important as *what* you eat. *Calories eaten in the morning will cause less weight gain than the same number of calories eaten later in the day.* People who work from 9 to 5 really shouldn't eat after 7 or 8 P.M. (to allow three to four hours before retiring). The CEOs in my study eat dinner at about 7 P.M.

The following formula will help you figure the exact amount of calories for you to lose weight. Depending on your metabolism and gender, you may have to make initial adjustments in your caloric allowances and/or amount of exercise as you observe results. For example, people who have dieted a lot and women as a whole (sorry about that, ladies) will lose weight more slowly. Use this formula as you set up your program with the HWW Diet & Exercise Calendar.

CALORIES FOR MAINTAINING WEIGHT:

Current weight × 10 = Basal Metabolic Rate (BMR)

BMR × 1.3 or 1.5 or 2.0 = Daily Maintenance Calories (D.M.C.)

(1.3 = light activity; 1.5 = medium; 2.0 = heavy)

Example:

(120 pounds × 10) × 1.5 = 1,800 D.M.C. (to maintain 120 pounds if
your activity is medium)

CALORIES TO LOSE ONE TO TWO POUNDS PER WEEK

Here is how many calories you need to subtract to lose one
or two pounds per week:

One pound per week = subtract 500 calories from D.M.C.
Two pounds per week = subtract 1,000 calories from D.M.C.

When America's highest-ranked need to lose a few pounds,
most have evolved to the stage where they simply cut back portions
a little and eliminate fatty foods and desserts. Although it is currently
popular to count milligrams of fat, protein, carbohydrates, or sodium,
the men and women I interviewed generally do not get caught up in
that process. They just eat nutritiously. You, too, can do this—you
already know more about nutrition than you think. It doesn't have
to be complicated.

HOW TO OVERCOME BINGEING

To maintain control over your weight, you may have to conquer the binge demon. Bingeing causes a lose/gain cycle that is actually worse than gradual weight gain, because it can permanently
alter your metabolism and contribute to hardening of the arteries. If
that's not enough, the muscle tissue that is lost during too-rapid
weight loss is replaced with fat tissue during the gain phase, especially if you aren't exercising. No wonder dieting, as most people
know it, is so difficult. The HWW Diet & Nutrition Program conquers
the binge demon, in part, by desensitization (eating the foods you
have deprived yourself of, on a regular basis). The glamour of foods
quickly diminish when they are readily available and treated as com-
monplace. In my practice, clients are usually assigned binge foods to
be eaten daily, focusing on one food at a time. Each desensitization
period usually lasts one to three weeks.

One client habitually binged on pancakes, sabotaging his weight
loss program in the process. He finally revealed that as a child he
was denied pancakes because he was fat. I immediately assigned him
pancakes on a daily basis (shifting to whole wheat pancakes with
HWW Fruit Spread instead of butter and syrup). He loved it—and
ate them at least once a day for twelve consecutive days. The "pancake
mystique" is now gone from his life—and so are 46 pounds!

Allergy Foods.   Occasionally, you will find foods that you are sensitive to and cannot tolerate. This intolerance may be manifested by perpetual out-of-control eating of that food (it's sugar for me). I call these out-of-control foods *allergy foods* (as differentiated from binge foods). In my experience, an addiction to a specific food is commonly caused by an allergy to that food. Much as alcoholics are often allergic to an ingredient in alcohol (such as corn—a common allergy food), so can food addicts be allergic to a certain food (or food ingredient). The luckier food allergy victims break out in hives and simply can't tolerate the food. The less fortunate spend a lifetime fighting an uncontrollable craving for the food. I must mention that while the allergic/addicted relationship is not yet scientifically validated, I definitely consider it when treating the binge syndrome. In any case, when binge desensitization doesn't work and desire for the food continues to rage in an addictive manner, the best, and strangely enough, *easiest* solution, is complete abstinence. Stop playing with fire. Get the food out of your life, once and for all, as an alcoholic must deal with alcohol. Make it a one-time war instead of a lifetime of agonizing battles, and get on with your life. A good Trigger Statement (see page 100) to use here might be "I've got more important

---

The Keys to Binge Therapy

Stop the physical cravings

- Each day during Phase 1, incorporate the foods you have been denied into your diet. (If there are many, you may want to focus on one at a time.)
- Learn to separate binge foods from addictive foods (if, after a week, you can't control your portions, that food may be addictive).
- Use abstinence with addictive foods (apply Reprogram Your Thoughts, page 105).
- Tune into your mind/body connection and apply the Scanning Technique as described on page 104. Before you run to the refrigerator, sit down for 30 seconds to 5 minutes. Ask yourself where in your body you feel the discomfort of craving. Then focus on that area and relax into it; "surrender" to it. Explore the area with awareness and allow the discomfort to break up (it may or may not—don't try to force a result). Just be willing to "be" with it.

Stop the emotional cravings

- Examine your internal binge messages. Then work to eliminate the self-sabotaging behavior and build self-esteem. Read books such as John Bradshaw's *Healing the Shame that Binds You* for guidance and/or seek professional help.
- As with physical cravings, apply the scanning technique as described on pages 105–106 (Motivation, Step #9).

things to do with my life than constantly playing around with this thing."

Approximately 70 percent of my clients are successful with the binge desensitization method (reintroducing foods they have formerly denied themselves). Another 5 percent fall into the allergic/addictive food category. With the remaining 25 percent, it is necessary to consider the emotional aspect of their bingeing. Low self-esteem and a feeling of hopelessness, often accompanied by an abusive past (physical, emotional, and/or sexual), are commonly at the root of emotional bingeing. Healing the emotional causes of bingeing is important, because they affect self-sabotage in most *every* aspect of one's life.

How to Get Results: The Three Stages of The HWW Diet & Nutrition Program

The HWW Diet & Program has three key stages. Master one stage before moving on to the next stage. The stages, their goals, and what should happen during each one are as follows:

Stage 1—Goals: Eliminate Binges. Eat Foods That Taste Good. Limit Quantity.

The first step is to eliminate binges, as discussed earlier, if this is a problem for you. Then the fun part: You must eat foods that taste good. What's the tradeoff? Simple. *Quantity*. You must limit your intake. Remember, caloric intake and expenditure of calories are the bottom line in losing weight. (Refining of food *quality*, such as fat intake, comes next.) You are learning a very important lesson at this stage: how many calories are actually going into your mouth. Basic self-psychology and motivational principles are initiated during this stage.

Stage 2—Goals: Learn to Think Nutrition.

By Stage 2, counting calories should be second nature. You are now ready to add nutritional awareness to your program. Concentrate more on the quality of the food you eat—its nutritional value—while maintaining the "it must taste good" priority of Stage 1. In Stage 2, you will also practice some intermediate self-psychology and motivational principles.

Stage 3—Goals: Experiment and Refine.

In Stage 3, you are free to experiment and refine, so that you can add even more good tastes and nutrition, as well as greater variety, to your diet. Increasingly, in Stage 3 you become your own expert and motivator and can evolve accordingly. You will utilize advanced self-psychology and motivational principles.

> **Note:** The amount of time needed to go from one stage to the next may vary from person to person. Use the suggested timeline as a starting point. Record your goals and daily progress on your Personal Goals Chart, page 157 and on the HWW Diet and Exercise Calendar and/or the HWW HealthStyle Calendar, pages 164 and 165. *Be specific with your goals.*

STAGE 1

Weeks 1–7

1. Eat only foods that taste good.   Here is how to create your "Working Foods List":

   a. Make a list of all your favorite foods.

   b. Cross off any addictive (out of control) foods.

   c. Add the healthful foods you truly enjoy but don't consume often enough.

This is just the start of your ongoing Working Foods List. Try to stop eating the addictive foods, but don't be distressed if you slip. You will be working on avoiding these foods throughout your program. Steer your attention, instead, toward the healthful foods you enjoy and refer to the breakfast, lunch, and dinner suggestions previously discussed. Avoid the denial state of mind, and remember that you are *choosing* to improve your HealthStyle.

2. Limit Quantity.   Count and record calories, unless your personality rebels at the thought. Use the HWW Diet and Exercise Calendar on page 162. Learn where your calories are coming from and how many you are consuming. Calculate the number of calories you can have and still lose one to two pounds per week. (For women, the totals are about 1,000 to 1,200. For men, 1,800 to 2,000.) While all calories are not assimilated equally in the body (remember, fat calories are stored more easily than carbohydrate calories), counting calories is still the best way to start. More attention to *types* of calories is addressed next. If you decide not to count calories, apply the Evolutionary Approach (pages 216–217) by applying reasonable but specific limitations one at a time (for example, reducing certain foods, cutting out late-night eating or avoiding snacking). Be willing to experience hunger and think of it as "fat is burning" time.

3. Apply the Evolutionary Approach   (pages 216–217) as needed to help you ease habitual, unhealthful foods out of your life. Work on one food at a time, as you are ready.

My Working Foods List

My Favorite Foods:

(1)

(2)

(3)

(4)

(5)

(6)

(Now cross off any addictive (out of control) foods)

Healthful Foods I Will Add:

(7)

(8)

(9)

(10)

(11)

(12)

Healthful Foods I Would "Like to Like" (stage 3):

(13)

(14)

(15)

(16)

(17)

(18)

4. Eat alone in silence as much as possible. According to a Georgia University study, you eat for a longer period and up to 44 percent more food when you eat with others. Also, no reading, TV, or radio while eating. Apply the Scanning Technique (Motivating, Step #9, page 104). Learn to taste food and recognize the satisfied stage (the stage before full).

5. Implement Stage 1 Motivation principles   (page 212).

STAGE 2

Weeks 8–15

1. Put more focus on nutrition and the breakfast/lunch/dinner of Champions suggestions. Check your Working Foods List and mark out the non-healthful food(s) from "My Favorite Foods" that you can willingly reduce. Use your HWW calendars. Reduce only one food at a time. Continue to *apply the Evolutionary Approach* to help you through specific areas, such as reducing fats or refined carbohydrates. As you clean up your diet and guide your thinking in the direction of health, your taste buds will change. If paced and guided properly, evolution will become natural.

2. Stop recording calories when you feel ready (although many choose to keep ongoing records). Instead, simply estimate the number of calories in each meal. This helps establish a calorie-aware state of mind.

3. Continue Binge Therapy and Reprogramming Technique as needed. Keep applying Scanning Technique with meals.

4. Eat Early. We generally consume 60 percent of our calories after 6 P.M. Eat 75 percent of your calories before 1 P.M. and lose weight, or at least try not to eat late or to snack after dinner.

5. Implement Stage 2 Motivation principles   (page 212).

STAGE 3

Weeks 16–Forever

1. Expand your nutrition focus while keeping your diet interesting. Try to keep a jump on dietary boredom. Add to your "Working Foods List" any healthful foods you would "like to like" and experiment with creative ways to make them delicious. Also consult cookbooks and visit health-food stores and restaurants for ideas. Also see the HWW Recipes in Chapter 11 for more ideas. Here is an example of how to keep salads interesting. Find or make a good salad dressing and use ingredients you know you like or try new ones, such as peas, shredded jicama, chicken, feta cheese. Another helpful tip: Build separate "Working Foods Lists" for breakfast, lunch, and dinner. List your favorite healthful meal choices that you have developed over the past sixteen weeks. These lists can serve as healthful meal reminders and can help you get back on track during stale periods, such as after the holidays or after returning from trips.

2. Stop counting calories (when you feel ready). Allow a global awareness of food to develop, encompassing good taste, nutrition, calories, and *choice*. Let your experience guide you.

3. Apply the Reprogramming and the Evolutionary Approach as needed.

4. Implement Stage 3 Motivation principles   (page 212).

5. Revert to Stage 1 and Stage 2 eating principles when needed.   Occasional dietary slips or dips in motivation will occur. Expect them and try to avoid them, but be willing to take a half step back in your program to refresh your motivation.

6. Keep using your Personal Goals Calendar.

THE EVOLUTIONARY APPROACH TO HEALTHFUL EATING

While Binge Therapy can desensitize you to foods of which you have been deprived, the Evolutionary Approach can be used to ease commonly eaten, unhealthful foods out of your life.

The value and effectiveness of taking the Evolutionary Approach, when shifting from a lifestyle to a HealthStyle, cannot be emphasized enough. Forcing a program, taking on too much too soon, or doing something incorrectly can ruin an otherwise good program and actually jeopardize your health and motivation. Instead, enjoy the process and just take one thing at a time.

Everyone entering the HWW HealthStyle Program starts from a different place and has different weaknesses, strengths and goals. One person may want to work on cutting down on sweets while another may want to work on whittling down red meat consumption. The next section will take you through a sample Evolutionary Plan that is designed to help you refine your diet. It will enable you to get from donuts to oatmeal (or whatever your goal) as painlessly as possible. It also shows you how any diet should slowly evolve.

Two common types of food abuse are described here. If you don't fit into either category, but simply want to improve your current diet, study the plan and adapt it to your specific dietary goals and needs. The point is to set a *REASONABLE* but *SPECIFIC* limit for yourself in whatever area you are trying to improve. Don't start a new goal until you are comfortable with the current one. Use your HWW calendars to help you implement your own Evolutionary Plan.

Carboholics Versus Fataholics

Two common types of food abusers can be categorized as Sweet/Carboholics and Salty/Fataholics. Sweet/Carboholics love refined carbohydrates and sweets and could gladly forgo a meal for bread, sweets, and junk food. "Carbohydrate loading" to them means loading up on chocolate chip cookies, donuts, bread, and chips. Meat is not a priority for Sweet/Carboholics. In fact, many of these people give vegetarians a bad name. They realized somewhere along the line that they had inadvertently traded in meat for sugar/refined carbohydrates and were thrilled to discover a respectable title (vegetarian) to cover for their poor eating habits.

Fataholics, on the other hand, choose fatty and/or salty foods—preferably in the form of two to three "hot squares" a day. Their claim to fame is that in regard to refined carbohydrates, they can "take it or leave it." They don't eat many desserts or snacks and may even heroically skip breakfast or lunch. The Fataholics' favorite foods include salty and/or fatty foods such as red meat, chips, cheese, heavy sauces, pizza, hamburgers, nuts, cold cuts. Ice cream, high in fat, is a popular choice when a sweet is craved. (Ice cream also fills the bill for Carboholics—no wonder it is America's most popular dessert.)

If you are a Carboholic or a Fataholic, permanent weight loss will not happen until you clean up your diet. You must remove or at least reduce the foods from your diet that are jeopardizing your weight loss (and health). As they are eliminated, weight loss will start occurring naturally. Why? Because once the body becomes nutritionally balanced, it no longer sends out inappropriate demands for second helpings and junk foods. When you have comfortably reduced or eliminated these foods, you can concentrate even more on weight loss.

Sample Evolutionary Schedules

Note: Chart your Evolutionary goals and progress on your HWW calendars (pages 162–165). Be specific.

Carboholics

CARBOHOLICS: Weeks 1–7

1. Junk breakfasts/donuts: Substitute a healthful break-fast (such as a HWW Muffin or whole wheat toast with all-fruit spread) for a junk breakfast at least *once a week* and gradually but specifically *increase the number of healthful breakfasts to three to four days per week.*

2. Snacks: One sweet snack per day is okay, such as one candy bar, two cookies, one piece of pie or cake. Gradually replace other sweet snacks with allowable snacks such as rice cakes, fruit, raw vegetables, popcorn, or raw nuts.

3. Dessert: One dessert per day. Or, if bread is your weak spot, set a reasonable but specific limit for yourself (one notch lower than your norm).

Tips: If you usually don't snack on sweets, don't start now. On the other hand, if it's asking too much to give up your morning donut right now, wait until you're ready. In other words, adapt this plan to meet *reasonable* but *specific* guidelines suited to your needs. Start experimenting with exchanging fruit and fruit-sweetened snacks as part of your daily sweet allowance.

CARBOHOLICS: Weeks 8–15

1. Junk breakfast: Two per week.

2. Snacks: Three sweets per week.

3. Desserts: Four desserts per week, weeks 8–11, and three desserts per week, weeks 12–15. Experiment with healthful substitutes as part of your dessert allowance.

Tips: Don't keep sweets in the house (go out for them each time). Try substituting homemade, oil-free muffins (see Recipes, Chapter 11) for store-bought muffins and save 100 to 200 calories each time. Eat whole-grain rye crackers versus the overprocessed variety. Have a bagel instead of a croissant. Have cold cereal or oatmeal instead of store-bought granola. Eat an English muffin (whole wheat) instead of a fast-food roll or biscuit.

CARBOHOLICS: Weeks 16–Forever

1. Junk breakfasts: One per week.

2. Snacks: One to two sweets a week.

3. Desserts: No dinner desserts (fruit as evening snack is okay). Two lunch desserts per week okay. Experiment with healthful substitutes.

Fataholics

FATAHOLICS: Weeks 1–7

1. Red meat, butter, or other dietary weak spot. Reduce to reasonable but specific amount. Example: cut red meat meals from seven to four per week.

2. Snacks: One salty, fatty snack per day, but you are not allowed to keep them in the house.

3. Dessert: One per day (ice cream or other fatty treat) if desserts are a problem area.
Tips: Add healthful "treats." For example, put a basket of fresh fruit on the top shelf of refrigerator; or go out for frozen yogurt.

FATAHOLICS: Weeks 8–15

1. Red meat or other weak spot: Three servings a week.

2. Snacks: Four (fatty, salty) snacks per week.

3. Dessert: Four desserts, weeks 8–11, and three desserts, weeks 12–15.
Tips: Try substituting all-bean chili for all-meat chili; eat turkey hot dogs instead of beef (save 45 fat-laden calories); eat plain bean burritos versus beef and cheese burritos (save 200 calories); use yogurt instead of sour cream; eat plain cheese or no-cheese pizza instead of "the works" (blot off excess oil, too) and save 100 to 250 calories.

FATAHOLICS: Weeks 16–Forever

1. Red meat: One to two (on occasion) servings a week. Eventually eliminate all (except occasional) processed sandwich meats, sausage, bacon, corned beef and other meat.

2. Snacks: One to two per week.

3. Desserts: No dinner desserts. Two lunch desserts per week.
Tip: As you become comfortable with each Evolutionary level, select another problem area to go after, as you are ready, such as red meat, processed meats, high-fat milk, cheese, chips.

DON'T DEPRIVE

Chapter Eleven

THE HWW SPEED COOKING PLAN

You can't perform if you're not healthy. You can't keep up the pace.

—David Miller, J. C. Penney

YOUR MASTER PLAN TO GOOD EATING

Run your kitchen like a business, and your body will evidence your efforts.

Whether you run a major corporation or a household, you are the only one who can take full responsibility for what goes into your mouth. That responsibility includes foods you "encounter" while traveling, in restaurants, as well as at home. Don't panic, however, and think you must become a five-star health-food chef to become svelte. It's all quite easy. In fact, many aspects of your eating plan can even be delegated. The point is not to underestimate this part of your HealthStyle. Bad eating habits are the weak link in most programs, and educated eating is the only thing that can strengthen this link.

The Speed Cooking Plan presented in this chapter and the next will help you coordinate all aspects of your eating—from stocking your kitchen to shopping, cooking, and even "eating on the run" during hectic days. The Speed Cooking Plan is a new concept designed for today's Era of Hurry that affects your whole life. This plan is a time-efficient approach designed to provide meals that are quick, low in calories, nutritious, and best of all, delicious. Most important, it is doable. *It is meant for men and women who want to eat well but can't devote their lives to it.* The Speed Cooking Plan is more about how to cook than about how to follow a recipe. It's more about how to get a tasty nutritious meal out fast rather than mastering complex cooking skills.

By following this system, you can eat like a king (or CEO) with minimal effort. If you want to put forth *no* effort, and if you have no spouse to provide the necessary labor, consider hiring someone to shop and cook, just as you would to clean your house or do your laundry. Man (or woman) cannot, or at least *should* not, live on restaurant food alone.

Anyone serious about achieving maximum performance with minimum effort can benefit from the Speed Cooking Plan. It can help your life—and your body—run a lot more smoothly.

Meal Stocking: Cook It Now—Eat for a Week.   The Speed Cooking Plan is based on the concept of cooking and shopping just once a week to create a supply of food to last you the whole week as well as to establish an ongoing freezer stock. The art of "freezer recruiting," that is, planning meals around your freezer reserve, will save you the inconvenience of daily meal preparation. You will quickly appreciate that having healthful, ready-to-eat meals in the freezer is like having money in the bank.

Multiway Recipes.   In addition, the Speed Cooking Plan shows you how to cook several different meals simultaneously, creating variations from a basic recipe. HWW Multiway Recipes include Multiway chicken, soup, rice, beans, muffins, and even salad.

HOW TO COOK FAST AND SMART: RECIPES FOR SUCCESS

According to William Castelli, M.D., director of the Framingham Heart Study, most Americans eat a diet consisting of only about ten recipes. Unfortunately, most of the foods in these ten recipes are not very healthful. Castelli says that rather than overwhelm ourselves with the science of nutrition, we should put a little thought into finding ten new, healthful meals. Naturally, we should also keep ourselves updated on dietary advice and follow it. Exchanging any or all of your ten most-consumed meals for the meals described in this book can make a painless—in fact, pleasurable and positive—change in favor of your health and longevity. Your meals can become a health "plus" instead of a "minus."

The following recipes include a few favorite originals from the HWW leaders themselves, along with my tried-and-true favorites that have helped create new "Ten Most Wanted" lists for my clients. The best news? These recipes are designed to be delicious as well as *simple*, so that *ANY*one can follow them.

Easy directions and few ingredients are used in these recipes. Long ago, I quit following fixed recipes, after repeated episodes of frantic but futile last-minute, kitchen-torn-apart-in-preparation searches for various missing ingredients. There I was, left staring at a full color, good-enough-to-eat glossy photo of the finished product, mouth watering, stomach growling. It is from those past frustrations that I designed the following recipes to have a lot of flexibility. The idea is to learn to ad lib and *keep going* if you don't have every ingredient listed. Some people like to pick a rainy day and turn their kitchen into a veritable food factory, making several recipes at once. Others prefer to keep their freezer stocked by doubling or tripling recipes as they go.

These recipes make large enough "stocking" quantities for one or two people. If you have a large freezer or more than two people to feed, you may want to make larger amounts. Incidentally, it's a good idea to label your freezer stock with masking tape and keep an ongoing Freezer Chart (taped to the inside of a nearby cupboard) which can keep you updated as to what goes in to and out of your freezer.

If you are new to cooking, *DON'T BE AFRAID OF THE KITCHEN*. Start with the following recipes and allow yourself to get braver and more creative as you go. Experiment to suit personal taste and learn to improvise using the ingredients you have on hand. You will see how the recipes all work together in the Menu Planning section.

Chevron's James Sullivan loves to cook creatively and has "a dozen different ways to do chicken." He bones and skins his own, experiments with various ingredients, and usually broils his chicken. Some of his personal favorite recipes are Chicken with Louisiana Pepper Sauce, Chicken with Lemon (and a "dab" of butter) and Chicken with capers. Sorry, no repeatable recipes. He just grabs and creates with his mood. Christian Dior's Colombe Nicholas says that cooking actually helps her reduce stress. Cooking offers a creative outlet and can impart a sense of accomplishment.

The following Recipe Index can help you organize and plan your meals.

RECIPE INDEX

Multiway Chicken and Rice: Pages 228–231

Fish: Pages 231–232

Multiway Rice: Pages 232–234

Vegetables: Pages 234–236

"Mayo," Sour Cream, Salad Dressings: Pages 237–238

Salads: Pages 238–241

Beans: Pages 241–242

Soups: Pages 243–246

Stocks and Salty Flavorings
Multiway Bean/Pea Soup
       Lentil Soup
       Split Pea
       Black Bean
       Hot Black Bean Soup
       Dahl ("Gravy")
Chicken (or Turkey) Soup
Curried (or Plain) Creamed Vegetable Soup
Vegetable Soup

Pasta: Pages 246–247

Pasta Primavera

Bread, Muffins, Cereal, Yogurt Milk, Fruit Spread: Pages 247–251

Multiway Muffins or Breads
Bread
Shepherds Granola (raw, wheat-free)
Yogurt Milk
Fruit Spread or Dessert, Yogurt Tricks

Desserts/Snacks: Pages 251–253

Randy's Go-Juice
Paula Kent Meehan's Five-Minute Pie
Frozen Nutty Bananas
Frozen Grapes
Frozen Yogurt

MULTIWAY CHICKEN AND RICE

Here are four chicken and rice recipes that are very much alike, yet are deliciously different, and can be made simultaneously and frozen for future enjoyment. The chicken does not have to be breast meat, and it doesn't have to be boned. Ask your butchers to let you know when they have a sale and have them skin your chicken—it's a real time saver. Important note: Depending on your preference or need, the chicken can be: (1) precooked (boiled) and then added to recipes (for a quicker reheat), or (2) added to recipes while raw and/or frozen and put back in the freezer. Reheating works quite well with these dishes, since there is plenty of moisture in the recipes to keep the chicken moist, even with freezing. But if you are going to reheat already-cooked chicken, undercook it slightly the first time. Another time-saver: Mix up the basic rice/yogurt/Vege-Sal mixture (about 5 parts rice to 1 part yogurt) and divide to customize for each recipe (omit the yogurt and Vege-Sal (herbal salt mixture) for Chicken Pilaf and Chicken, Rice, and Veggies as indicated). Make up your own variations. Serve one tonight and freeze the others for future instant meals.

CHICKEN AND RICE PICANTE

8–10 skinned, boned chicken breasts (or 6 whole legs, etc.),
   3 pounds total
4 cups cooked brown rice
3/4 cup medium hot Mexican salsa
3/4 cup plain nonfat yogurt
1-1/2 teaspoons Vege-Sal (herbal salt mixture)
1/2 cup (2 oz) shredded low-fat cheese or 5 tablespoons dry
   Parmesan

To prepare this dish, proceed as follows:
1. Boil chicken 30 minutes (or use undercooked or raw chicken and cook recipe longer when heating to eat).
2. Place chicken in casserole pan (or pans, depending on recipe size).
3. Mix together other ingredients, except cheese.
4. Pour mixture over chicken.
5. Sprinkle with cheese.

Bake:
350 degrees for 35 minutes, covered. (350 degrees for 1 hr. if heating from freezer, chicken precooked. 350 degrees for up to 1 1/2

hours if heating from freezer, chicken uncooked. Cut into chicken occasionally to check doneness.)

Calories:

315 calories per serving. 12 servings
(1 serving = 4 oz. chicken, 1/3 cup rice)

Tips:

- Cook enough to provide three to four meals (reheated) for the week.
- Label extra dishes and freeze.
- Vege-Sal. This is a nice herb-salt combination by Modern Products that is sold nationwide. If you use plain salt, use only half as much.
- Use pan sizes that suit your needs. You may want to freeze some in smaller cooking containers (8″ × 8″) or even in single serving sizes. Many prefer making one large serving (9-1/2 × 13-1/2 container) for themselves to eat hot or cold for a few days or for entertaining (it's quite a treat to come home from work, toss something from freezer to oven, and spend your time on other party preparations).
- Buy salsa at a health food store or use Pace brand from the grocery store. It has no sugar or preservatives. Use no-salt salsa if you have high blood pressure.
- Boil enough chicken to freeze for other recipes such as soups, Chinese rice, salad, or sandwiches. (Cut up the extra chicken and put in freezer bags.)
- Cool chicken stock (water the chicken was boiled in), skim off fat, and freeze in plastic containers or freezer bags. Use later as soup stock or to cook with. For example, "stir fry" with chicken stock rather than with oil, or use chicken stock to make rice. Chicken stock adds taste to recipes but also adds nutrients, particularly amino acids, which can help the immune system. There's some truth to the old saying, "Eat chicken soup when you're sick."

CHICKEN AND RICE CURRY

8–10 skinned, boned chicken breasts (or 6 whole legs, etc.),
    3 pounds total
4 cups cooked brown rice
3/4 cup frozen peas (not thawed)
3/4 cup plain nonfat yogurt
1-1/2 tablespoons curry powder
1/8 cup (or more) raisins
1-1/2 teaspoons Vege-Sal

1. Boil chicken 30 minutes (or use undercooked or raw chicken and cook recipe longer when heating to eat).
2. Place chicken in casserole pan(s).
3. Mix together other ingredients.
4. Pour mixture over chicken.
5. See Chicken Picante Tips.

Heat:

350 degrees for 35 minutes, covered. (Or cook 1 hour if heating from freezer with chicken precooked. Cook up to 1-1/2 hours if using from freezer with chicken uncooked. Cut into chicken occasionally to check doneness.)

Calories:

290 calories per serving. 12 servings.
(1 serving = 4 oz. chicken, 1/3 cup rice)

Tip:

For festive meals, serve with Indian condiments—crushed peanuts, banana pieces, chutney, shredded coconut. Also, serve with Raita (HWW Cucumber Salad for an authentic Indian meal).

CHICKEN PILAF

8–10 skinned, boned chicken breasts (or 6 whole legs, etc.),
   3 pounds total
4 cups cooked brown rice
4 tablespoons tamari (second choice—soy sauce)
1-1/2 tablespoons sunflower seeds, sliced almonds, and/or pine nuts

Optional:
sliced mushrooms
green onions

1. Boil chicken 30 minutes (or use undercooked or raw chicken and cook recipe longer when heating to eat).
2. Place chicken in large casserole pan(s).
3. Mix together other ingredients.
4. Pour mixture over chicken.
5. See Chicken Picante tips.

Heat:
350 degrees for 35 minutes covered. (Or cook 1 hour if heating from freezer with chicken precooked. Cook up to 1-1/2 hours if

using from freezer with chicken uncooked. Cut into chicken to check doneness.)

Calories:
285 per serving. 12 servings.
(1 serving = 4 oz. chicken, 1/3 cup rice)

CHICKEN, RICE, AND VEGGIES

8–10 skinned, boned chicken breasts (or 6 whole legs, etc.),
   3 pounds total
4 cups cooked brown rice
2 cups mixed vegetables (not thawed)*
1-1/2 teaspoons Vege-Sal

*Note:
Fresh vegetables are preferable, if you have them on hand. But keep frozen vegetables stocked for a quick, healthful, emergency meal.

1. Boil chicken 30 minutes (or use undercooked or raw chicken and cook recipe longer when heating to eat).
2. Place chicken in large casserole pan(s).
3. Mix together other ingredients.
4. Pour mixture over chicken.
5. Sprinkle with onions and almonds before serving.
6. See Chicken Picante tips.

Heat:
350 degrees for 35 minutes, covered. (Or cook 1 hour if heating from freezer with chicken precooked. Cook up to 1-1/2 hours if using from freezer with chicken uncooked.) Cut into chicken to check doneness.

Calories:
285 calories per serving. 12 servings
(1 serving = 4 oz. chicken, 1/3 cup rice)

FISH

Basic Tips:
• Buy fresh fish and cook it the same day or the next at the latest.
• If freezing is a must, put fish in a long, flat plastic container, cover with milk and freeze (takes away "fishy" taste when thawed). Don't ask me about the wasted milk.

- POACHED: Cover large saucepan with 1/4 inch water and 1 teaspoon lemon juice. Sprinkle with basil, dill or other favorite herb. Experiment. Turn heat on medium-high and poach, turning over once, until fish flakes when tested with a fork and is no longer pink in the middle (5 to 7 minutes).
- GRILLED: Use special hand held fish-grill (inexpensive) or put fish in aluminum foil. Poke holes in top and bottom and put on charcoal grill. Cook until it flakes, as in Step 3. Great taste.
- Improvise. If you don't love the pure taste of fish, try it Mexican style (with salsa in pan), teriyaki style (with teriyaki in pan), etc. Experiment.

Calories:
100–250 calories per 4 oz. serving (depending on fish)

MULTIWAY RICE

Rice is a wonderful addition to your freezer stock. It is handy to have a variety of rice dishes available to add to any meal. Following is the basic rice recipe for plain rice, followed by five variations. Most are take-offs on the Multiway Chicken recipes, so they could be made at the same time. Or you can just make a big batch of rice and divide to make any or all of the following dishes.

RICE

(For making your own customized amounts, proportions are
    always 1:2, rice to water)
3 cups brown rice
6 cups water

1. Add together and bring to a boil.
2. Reduce heat to simmer (lowest setting).
3. Cover and let simmer until small "craters" dot surface (30 to 45 minutes).

Makes:
8 to 9 cups cooked rice

Calories:
100 calories per 1/2 cup

Tips:
- Use 6 cups of chicken stock (the water used to boil the chicken) instead of water or use sodium-free, store-bought stock, or vegetable stock (water from steamed vegetables).

- Add 1 teaspoon of dried basil or other favorite herb to plain rice recipe for added flavor.
- To freeze rice, use resealable plastic bags that can be defrosted quickly in the microwave. Use smaller ones for one person, larger ones for the family or groups.

MULTIWAY Rice Variations:

1. MEXICAN RICE

Per 4 cups cooked rice add:

1/2 cup Mexican salsa
1-1/2 teaspoons Vege-Sal

2. INDIAN CURRY RICE

Per 4 cups cooked rice add:

1-1/2 tablespoons curry
1-1/2 teaspoons Vege-Sal
3/4 cup frozen (not thawed) peas
1/8 cup raisins

3. CHINESE RICE

Per 4 cups cooked rice add:

3 tablespoons Liquid Aminos or tamari (natural "soy sauce")
Optional—For a complete Chinese meal, add all or any of the following:
1 can water chestnuts, sliced, and/or bamboo shoots
1 stalk celery, cut into 1/2-inch pieces
1/2 cup pea pods
1/4 red pepper, diced
1/2 cup broccoli flowerettes
1 cup sliced chicken (from the sliced chicken supply in the freezer)

1. Stir-fry all vegetables in saucepan for 2 to 5 minutes with Liquid Aminos and 1/8 inch water covering bottom of pan.
2. Add cooked rice and stir until heated through.
3. To serve: place on plate and sprinkle with a few raw peanuts, slivered almonds, or cashews.

4. RICE PILAF

Per 4 cups cooked rice add:

4 tablespoons tamari (second choice—soy sauce)
1-1/2 tablespoons sunflower seeds, sliced almonds, and/or pine nuts

Optional:
sliced mushrooms
green onions

Tip:
- For a quick solo dish, just add one tablespoon tamari, one teaspoon seeds/nuts per one cup of rice. Also, learn to toss in what you have and create a new dish each time.

5. RICE & VEGGIES

Per 4 cups cooked rice add:
2 cups frozen (not thawed) or fresh mixed vegetables
1-1/2 teaspoons Vege-Sal

- Heat rice and vegetables together in pan with 1/8 inch water.

VEGETABLES

STEAMED VEGETABLES

(Any or all of the following and any others you like):
Carrots
Red potatoes
Red cabbage
Broccoli
Cauliflower
Zucchini
Yams

1. Wash and slice (or break up) into small pieces.
2. Place in steamer over boiling water and cover.
3. Steam for 6 to 9 minutes.

Calories:
40 calories per 1/2-cup serving

Tips:
- Serve plain over rice, sprinkled with grated lowfat cheese, slivered almonds, and/or salad dressing.
- Use nonaluminum, two-pot-type steamer.
- Put "harder" vegetables, such as carrots, on the bottom (to cook faster).

COLOMBE'S GINGERED CARROTS

(A favorite dish of Christian Dior's president emeritus, Colombe Nicholas)

5–6 carrots, diced
2 pieces candied ginger, crumbled or grated (or dried pineapple or papaya)
1 teaspoon butter (or ghee)
dash of cinnamon

1. Wrap carrots, ginger and butter in heavy-duty aluminum foil.

Bake:
350 degrees, 30–60 minutes; the longer the more "candied" they get.

Calories:
40 calories per 1/2 cup serving

Tip:
I took the liberty of adapting Colombe's recipe to my cupboard. Dried papaya or pineapple works great in place of ginger. Ghee is a more healthful alternative to butter.

BAKED POTATO WITH BROCCOLI

1 baked potato
1/2 cup steamed broccoli

Optional:
1/4 cup steamed fresh mushrooms
1 tablespoon low-fat cheese, grated
HWW Salad Dressing

1. Bake potato (microwave or cook in oven at 375 degrees, 1 hour)
2. Cut potato in half lengthwise and mash both sides.
3. Cover with broccoli, mushrooms, cheese, and dressing.

Calories:
175 per potato without cheese

Tips:
• Wash potato before baking and pierce with knife or fork to create holes (so potato won't explode in oven).
• Eat the skin—it's good for you.

TWICE-BAKED POTATOES

6 baked potatoes (baked at 450 degrees for last 10 minutes to make
   skin stiff)
2 steamed zucchini squash, carrots, or yellow squash (or some of
   each)
1/4 onion chopped, steamed, or 1/4 cup dried onion flakes
1/2 cup nonfat milk or yogurt milk
1 teaspoon basil
3/4 teaspoon Vege-Sal (salt flavoring)

Optional:
1/4 cup grated low-fat cheese
1 teaspoon chives

1. Cut baked potatoes in half, lengthwise.
2. Hollow out insides leaving stiff potato skin shell.
3. Puree potato insides in food processor with other ingredients,
   except cheese.
4. Pour mix into potato skins and sprinkle with cheese.
5. Place on cookie sheets and put in freezer (uncovered) until
   frozen.
6. Wrap individually in ready-to-heat wrapping (plastic wrap for
   microwave, aluminum foil for oven), label, and store in freezer.

Calories:
80 calories per half potato

Tip:
This is easy to make simultaneously with Creamed Cauliflower
Soup.

YAMS

(Sweet and delicious. Great hot—or cold as dessert.)
1. Place washed yams on foil and/or cookie sheet and bake at 350
   degrees until skin is "baggy" (about two hours).
2. Cut open and serve (add nothing).

Calories:
160 calories each yam

Tip:
Make extras to reheat, eat cold, or to use for pies, muffins, breads,
soups.

HWW MAYO, SOUR CREAM, SALAD DRESSING

MAYO

1 cup nonfat plain yogurt
1 teaspoon Dijon mustard (or more to taste)

• Mix together and keep in closed container labeled "Mayo."

Calories:
8 calories per tablespoon (versus 100 per regular mayonnaise)

Tip:
Use as mayo for tuna or chicken salad, sandwich spread, etc.

SOUR CREAM

2 cups nonfat plain yogurt
4 cloves garlic, minced
1/4 onion, grated
1 tablespoon fresh cilantro, chopped

• Mix ingredients together and keep in closed container labeled "Sour Cream."

Calories:
60 calories per 1/3 cup

Tips:
• Baked potato topping: add chives, if desired.
• Dip and spread: add other herbs (Basil, Dill) and use on crackers or as a vegetable dip.
• Mexican Dip: add (Pace brand) salsa and use as a tostada topping or dip and spread as above.

SALAD DRESSING

(Delicious! It adds the finishing touch to more than salads.)
1 bottle Paul Newman's Salad Dressing (16 oz.) (optional: pour out up to half of the oil)
1 bottle Bernstein's lo-cal (16 oz.) or 2 bottles Wishbone Dijon Vinaigrette lo-cal salad dressing (8 oz. each)

• Mix 2:1 (lo-cal to Newman's) or any other portion to taste.

Calories:

approximately 12 calories per teaspoon (less if less oil used)

Tips:

- Bernstein's lo-cal dressing is quite nice on its own, for a no-fuss "out of the bottle" dressing.
- Newman's uses olive oil, which is mostly monounsaturated and therefore preferable to polyunsaturated oils used by most other dressings. Newman's is not low in calories, however, so it helps to mix it with a low-calorie dressing.
- If you use the Wishbone, first squeeze the bottle to force the oil out. Then combine with Newman's.
- Remember, your food must taste good or you won't stay with it. A good salad dressing is an important part of your menu. It can dress up what might otherwise be an ordinary meal. Take a little time to establish a healthful low-calorie dressing that is delicious. It doesn't matter if it's homemade or bottled. Make/buy enough to stock up for a month or two, so you will always have it on hand. Keep refrigerated.

SALADS

MULTIWAY SALAD

1 head favorite lettuce (the darker the better), finely chopped or torn
2–3 large carrots grated finely
1/3 head purple cabbage finely chopped, and/or 1 beet grated coarsely

Optional:

cherry tomatoes
celery
mushrooms
zucchini or yellow squash
green, red, or yellow pepper
jicama
avocado
hard boiled eggs (use just the whites for less fat)

- Chop any optional ingredients finely and place all ingredients in large (6–8 quart) covered plastic container.

Calories:

Approximately 30 calories per cup

Tips:

- Put damp paper towel over salad before covering. This keeps it fresh.
- Tomatoes, mushroom, avocado, and hard-boiled eggs don't keep well. Wait until just before serving to slice. However, they can be kept right in salad container (on top) for convenience.
- This salad can be made on Sunday and will last you most of the week.

Other uses for Multiway Salad throughout the week:

1. BEAN TOSTADA
1/4 cup vegetarian refried beans (no animal fat)
2 tablespoons grated low-fat cheese
Salad dressing and/or salsa

Optional:
tostada shell, tortilla, or blue corn chips

1. Heat beans.
2. Pour over tostada shell/tortilla or corn chips (optional).
3. Cover beans with Multiway Salad
4. Top with salad dressing and/or salsa and cheese.

Calories:
240 calories without tortilla/shell. One serving.

2. POTATO TOSTADA
- Slice open and mash one baked potato.
- Top with Multiway Salad and/or 1/4 avocado, 1/4 cup refried beans, salad dressing, HWW Sour Cream, salsa.

Calories:
285 with avocado, salad, and dressing

3. RICE TOSTADA
- Heat 1/2 cup HWW Mexican rice or plain rice.
- Top with Multiway Salad and/or 1/4 avocado, 1/4 cup refried beans, salad dressing, Multiway Sour Cream, salsa.

Calories:
280 with avocado, salad, and dressing

4. PLAIN LETTUCE SUBSTITUTE FOR SALAD

5. TUNA, CHICKEN, OR TURKEY SALAD

1 can tuna, chicken, or turkey (6 1/2 oz. can, in water)
1/8 cup HWW "Mayo" (more or less, depending on your tastes)
Vege-Sal to taste

Optional:
1/4 cup celery, finely chopped
1/8 cup onion, finely chopped

1. Mix together.
2. Place on top of Multiway Salad.

Calories:
40 per 1/4 cup

Tuna/Chicken Salad Tip:
Also use in sandwiches (in pita, too), on crackers and rice cakes, or alone.

CARROT SALAD

(A great cholesterol fighter)
2 cups large carrots grated finely
1 cup unsweetened crushed pineapple (canned)
1/4 cup raisins
1/4 cup orange juice concentrate (from frozen—apple juice okay, too)

Optional:
1 tablespoon coconut, unsweetened, dried (a treat if your cholesterol is okay, although amount is negligible per serving)
1/3 cup pine nuts or slivered almonds

1. Mix together and eat with meals or as a dessert or sweet snack.

Calories:
42 calories per 1/3 cup

RAITA (CUCUMBER/YOGURT SALAD)

1 large cucumber, peeled, cubed, and seeded (if large seeds)
2 cups plain nonfat yogurt

4 cloves garlic, minced
1/4 onion, grated
1 tablespoon fresh cilantro, chopped

1. Add all ingredients except cucumber and let sit at least one hour.
2. Add cucumber and let sit one hour before serving.

Calories:
50 calories per 1/3 cup serving

Tips:
- This is an East Indian side dish that is particularly complementary with entrees that are hot, such as **HWW Chicken and Rice Curry** or the **Hot Black Bean Soup.**
- The cucumber can be added with the other ingredients, but will be a little less crisp, especially if left overnight.
- Omit the cucumber and you have the **HWW Sour Cream Recipe.** And, vice versa, if you have the Sour Cream recipe already on hand, you can add just a little cucumber for a last-minute dinner salad.

BEANS

Basic guide:

1. Proportions: 1:3 dry beans to water. For example, 1 cup dry beans to 3 cups water.
2. Bean preparation:
   - Add beans to boiling water (per recipe)
   - Bring to boil and cook again for 2 minutes.
   - Turn off heat and let stand for 1 hour.
   - Bring to boil again and then simmer until done (per recipe)

   Note: This method is said to produce less gas than the soak method and is also faster. (Soak method: Pour boiling water over beans to cover them and soak half day or overnight. Discard soaking water.)

3. Add a dash of cayenne, when recipes allow, for improved digestion and reduced gas-producing tendency.
4. Use cold beans in green salads or as a salad (for example, toss together black beans, green onions, red/green/yellow peppers, corn, and salsa). Cold beans hold their shape when cooked a little less.

5. Calories for 1/2 cup cooked beans, about 120–125 (Fat content is less than 0.7 gram.)

MULTIWAY BEAN HOT DISH

3 cups mixed beans (mung, soy, navy, white, black-eyed peas, lima, etc.) (Apply bean preparation as described above.)
1 cup lentils, barley, and/or rice (for every additional cup, add 2 cups water.)
12 cups water
1 onion
1 teaspoon basil
1/3 cup tamari, Quick Sip, or Liquid Aminos

Optional:
1 tablespoon canola oil, olive oil, or ghee
1 green pepper

1. Bring ingredients to a boil. Reduce heat to low.

Cook:
1-1/2 to 2 hours (or 20 minutes in pressure cooker) until beans are soft with a thick and gravylike consistency.

Calories:
135 per 1/2 cup

Multiway Bean Hot Dish Variations:
• This is a versatile dish. Use any combination of beans and lentils, depending on what you have on hand. Aside from being a delicious "complete protein" hotdish, you can also use this dish as dahl (gravy) over rice, pasta or potato. To make soup, add water.
• Use this as your core dish for the week and change the taste every night:

(1) Mexican—add salsa to taste and melted cheese on top
(2) Refried beans—add salsa and put in blender to mash beans. Make a tostada or serve with rice.
(3) Goulash—add mixed frozen vegetables
(4) Indian—add curry to taste

Soups

STOCKS AND "SALTY" FLAVORINGS

Keep stocked on stocks. This is the vitamin-laden juice/water from steamed vegetables or boiled chicken to be used as a base for soups; "stir frying" vegetables, chicken, etc; as the liquid for cooking rice and beans; and for most any liquid used in meal preparation. Store your stocks in the freezer.

For natural, chemical-free salt substitutes, try *Quick Sip* by Bernard Jensen (for bouillon concentrate or soup stock, salt free), *Liquid Aminos* by Bragg (for soup stock or "soy sauce"), or *Vege-Sal* (contains sea salt). Salt-free does not necessarily mean sodium-free, so check labels if you are on a sodium-restricted diet. All three salt alternatives are good to have on hand for various uses.

Multiway Bean/Pea Soup

Here is the basic recipe for Lentil Soup, with variations following. Use your imagination—the possibilities are endless. Try every bean on the shelf, mix them, flavor them differently (herbs, ethnic flavorings—cajun, Mexican, Italian, Indian, etc.). Get four pots going at the same time.

LENTIL SOUP

9 cups water (use water from steamed vegetables)
3 cups lentils
1 large carrot, chopped
1 large purple onion, chopped
1/4 cup Quick Sip (Bernard Jensen)
1/2 teaspoon thyme
1 teaspoon basil
1/2 teaspoon marjoram

1. Steam carrot and onion.
2. Puree steamed carrot and onion in blender with 1 cup of steamer water.
3. Add to pot with other ingredients and bring to boil.
4. Reduce heat to simmer.

Cook:

1-1/2 to 2 hours, simmer, lid partway off until beans are soft and soup thickens (or 20 minutes in pressure cooker)

Calories:

135 for 1/2 cup (approximately the same for the following bean soups)

Tips:
- If you don't have the exact herbs on hand, feel free to improvise.
- The soups will thicken more as they cool. Add more water when ready to reheat, if necessary.

Multiway Bean/Pea Soup Variations:

1. SPLIT PEA SOUP
Same recipe, exchanging green and/or yellow split peas for lentils. You can also mix with lentils. Just keep proportions the same.

2. BLACK BEAN SOUP
Same recipe, exchanging black beans for lentils.

3. HOT BLACK BEAN SOUP
- Puree #2 in blender.
- Add Mexican salsa (mild, medium or hot) to taste.
- To serve, top with a spoonful of plain nonfat yogurt.

4. DAHL ("GRAVY")
Heat above thickened soup without adding water, and you'll get a gravy sort of consistency. Pour over rice or potatoes for a delicious dish. Add tumeric, cumin, coriander to taste—1/4 teaspoon each per 6 cups dahl. This is an East Indian dish. (Puree in blender for finer consistency.)

CHICKEN (OR TURKEY) SOUP
10 cups chicken stock (part stock and part plain water okay)
4 cups cooked chicken, cut into bite-sized pieces
1/3 cup chopped green onion
2 carrots, sliced finely
2 cups cooked rice
2 stalks celery, finely diced
1 teaspoon basil
1/4 teaspoon sage
Vege-Sal (salt flavoring) to taste as serving (not when cooking)

- Add together and cook (low) until vegetables are tender (30–45 minutes).

Calories:
90 per cup

Tip:

1. Use chicken with bones (versus boned) for better-tasting stock.
2. It's okay to cook with fresh stock, but let it cool first and lift fat from surface before eating or reheating.

CURRIED (OR PLAIN) CREAMED VEGETABLE SOUP

5 cups water, chicken or vegetable stock
1 head cauliflower, broken into flowerettes
3 large carrots
1/2 onion
2 zucchini or yellow crookneck squash
2 large russet potatoes or 5 red potatoes
1 teaspoon basil (crushed in palm of hand)
3 1/2 teaspoons Vege-Sal (herbal salt mix)

For a more exotic flavor add:

1/2 teaspoon cumin
1/2 teaspoon cinnamon
3 teaspoons curry (for a curry soup)

1. Cut (big pieces okay) and steam all vegetables until soft (use water as your stock)
2. Puree vegetables (food processor or blender) except 1/3 head cauliflower
3. Combine in pot with herbs, water, and the other 1/3 head cauliflower (broken into small flowerettes)
4. Heat, sprinkle with chopped parsley and serve

Calories:

80 calories per cup

Tips:

1. Split recipe in half and add curry to one half. Or double the recipe and add curry to one half.
2. This is easy to make simultaneously with Twice Baked Potatoes
3. If you intend to freeze, puree all of the cauliflower, leaving no small flowerettes.

VEGETABLE SOUP

10 cups chicken or vegetable stock (or water, with 1/4 cup Quick Sip)
1/3 cup chopped green onion (any onion okay)

2 large carrots, sliced finely
1/2 cup uncooked barley, rice, or potatoes
2 stalks celery, finely diced
1/2 cup dry beans (mixed—green, mung beans, aduki beans, great
   northern, white beans, yellow split peas, black-eyed peas)
2 cups frozen mixed vegetables—peas, corn, lima beans
1 teaspoon basil
2 bay leaves
Vege-Sal

1. Cook barley and/or beans in stock for one hour, simmer.
2. Add remaining ingredients except frozen vegetables and cook
   (simmer) for 30–45 minutes. Add frozen vegetables at end just to
   heat (five minutes).

Calories:
75 per cup

Tip:
Leftover steamed vegetables can be used to thicken soup. Put in
blender with a little water to puree. Then add to main soup
mixture or improvise and make Pureed Vegetable Soup. Be
Creative!

Pasta

PASTA PRIMAVERA
1 package uncooked spiral pasta (whole wheat, spinach, etc.)
1 head broccoli, broken into flowerettes
1 head cauliflower, broken into flowerettes

Optional:
2 large carrots, finely sliced or grated
1 red and/or yellow pepper, diced or sliced in long pieces
1 package frozen peas
1 package feta cheese, broken into small pieces

1. Steam vegetables (harder ones on bottom) while you:
2. Cook pasta and strain.
3. Mix all ingredients together in large plastic container for
   refrigeration.
4. Serve over Multiway salad bed, if desired.
5. Top with salad dressing and Parmesan cheese, if desired.

Calories:
130 per cup without dressing

Tips:
- Don't steam peppers or peas. They will heat when mixed in.
- This dish can be eaten hot the first day and cold the next day. Delicious!
- This recipe survives freezing quite well, except for the cauliflower.

BREADS, MUFFINS, CEREAL, YOGURT MILK, FRUIT SPREAD

Multiway Muffins or Breads

Meal-in-a-Muffin.   Muffins are a valuable asset to any freezer reserve. As mentioned, they can be a nutritious emergency meal-on-the-run or packed for a preworkout snack. I have not seen a store-bought muffin that you can buy that has no oil, sugar, or honey, is lo-cal, and tastes good, so this is a recipe worthy of your time. I often opt for the bread version over the muffin, as it is a little faster. The recipe is exactly the same for muffins and breads. To make bread, you simply put the batter (a single recipe makes one loaf) into a bread pan and cook longer (35 minutes instead of 20).

The advantage of making your own muffins or bread is that you can customize them to your taste. Leave out the wheat if you are *allergic*, use oat bran and carrots if you are trying to *lower cholesterol*, add wheat bran if you have *constipation* problems, and add goodies to suit your particular tastes. Use white flour for half the flour requirements if you need to ease into healthier-tasting foods. However, try to gradually reduce the amount of white flour in your recipes over time. Make a quadruple batch, divide four or more ways (4 cups batter per Basic Recipe), and flavor differently. Grab a muffin or slice of bread from the freezer on your way out the door—they thaw quickly.

MULTIWAY MUFFIN/BREAD RECIPE

Basic recipe—wheat and oil free
2 cups flour (1 cup oat flour, 1 cup rice flour) [OR:] (1 cup wheat flour or whole wheat pastry flour, 1 cup rice flour) [OR:] 1 cup oat bran (Use wheat bran if you have elimination problems), 1 cup flour (any)
1 cup applesauce

4 egg whites (or 2 eggs)
1/2 cup Yogurt Milk (see recipe) or nonfat milk
2 teaspoons baking powder
1 teaspoon baking soda
2 teaspoons vanilla
1/4 cup apple juice concentrate (undiluted frozen apple juice)
1/2 teaspoon Barleymalt Sweetener (optional)
2 teaspoons All-Spice or cinnamon (optional)

- Mix all ingredients together and place in nonstick muffin baking tins, or in a bread pan to make bread (a single recipe makes one loaf).

Bake:
400 degrees 18–20 minutes for muffins; 35–40 minutes for bread.
Makes 16 muffins or 16 slices of bread.

Calories:
67 calories each (if half bran) 76 calories each (if all flour)

MULTIWAY MUFFIN SUBSTITUTIONS

Substitute for equal amounts of flour (dry) or milk (liquid) or applesauce (sweetener):

Dry Ingredients:

1 cup oat flakes
1 cup Shepherd's Granola
1 cup oat or wheat bran

Liquid Ingredients:

1 cup nonfat plain yogurt
1/2 cup orange or apple juice concentrate (from frozen)

Sweeteners:

1 cup mashed banana, canned pumpkin, cooked yam, or sweet potato
1 cup crushed pineapple

MULTIWAY MUFFIN ADDITIONS

Sweeteners:

1 cup finely chopped apple, pear, and/or peach
1–2 cups finely shredded carrots and/or zucchini

1 cup blueberries (frozen okay)
1/2 cup raisins (white ones are nice), chopped dates, or prunes

Other:

1/2 cup chopped walnuts, sunflower seeds, etc.

Tips:
- Use 1 cup white flour in place of 1 cup of wheat, rice or oat flour if you need to ease into healthier-tasting foods. Over time, try gradually to reduce the amount of white flour.
- Use raisins with carrots in rice/oat flour recipe for a good taste.
- Beat eggs and fold in at the end for lighter muffins.
- Use nonstick muffin tins or paper muffin liners from grocery store.
- HWW Fruit Spread is a delicious, lo-cal spread for muffins or breads.

BREAD

Search high and low for the tastiest, most nutritious brand and load up your freezer. Preferably buy at a health food store. Don't let price or calories be your guide. Remember, half a slice of good hearty bread will satisfy much better than ten slices of a skinny little tasteless brand. If you have the time and desire to bake bread, great, but there are a lot of good ones out there, too. Isn't that an easy "recipe"?

SHEPHERD'S GRANOLA (RAW, WHEAT-FREE)

If you pick just one recipe to make, try this one. You can't buy an equivalent that is wheat-free (if desired), honey-free, unbaked (which reduces calories and rancidity), and is customized to your taste and need. You can practically live on it—it is great as an emergency meal or snack. If you have problems with constipation use wheat bran in place of oat bran; if you have an allergy to wheat (quite common) or want to lower your cholesterol, use more rice and oat bran; if you need both, use both. Tip: Rice bran is great for lowering cholesterol but has more of a "taste" than oat bran. Go easy at first. If you have trouble digesting raw foods, let the cereal soak in its milk for a few minutes before you eat it. This recipe is unbelievably easy and will last you "forever," especially if you double the recipe.

8 cups oat flakes (2 lbs.)
6 cups oat, rice, or wheat bran
6 cups barley flakes (1-1/2 lbs.)

3 cups rye flakes
2 cups chopped or slivered almonds
1 cup raisins (and/or chopped dates, dried apples, pineapple, etc.)
8 tablespoons cinnamon
1-1/2 tablespoons Barleymalt Sweetener (powdered)

Optional:
1/2 cup coconut, dried unsweetened (A treat if cholesterol isn't a
    problem. However, amount per serving is negligible.)

• Mix all ingredients together in large soup pots or mixing bowls.
  Store in plastic bags or plastic containers in refrigerator or
  freezer.

Calories:
137 calories per 1/3 cup

Tip:
Don't use the wheat bran if you don't need it. We get enough
wheat in our diets.

YOGURT MILK

*(For the calorie-conscious or milk-sensitive or those who want to
delete milk from their diets.)*
4 cups water
1 cup nonfat plain yogurt
1/8 teaspoon Barleymalt Sweetener (powdered)

1. Put yogurt and 2 cups water and sweetener in blender for 30
   seconds.
2. Add to other 2 cups of water and keep in bottle in refrigerator.
3. Give bottle a little shake before each use.

Note:
Make more or less if you wish—the ratio is 1:4 yogurt to water.
Barleymalt/sweetener to taste.

Calories:
8 calories per 1/3 cup serving

Tip:
• If you replace your nonfat milk with Yogurt Milk, you will save
  yourself at least three pounds' worth of calories per year.

- Many people past the age of 25 have some level of allergy to milk. Yogurt provides valuable stabilizing bacteria (for the intestines, etc.) as well as vitamin B12 (important to vegetarians).
- If you sweeten the Yogurt Milk enough, you will not need to add more sweetener when using with cereal.

FRUIT SPREAD OR DESSERT

1 cup nonfat plain yogurt
1-1/2 tablespoons all-fruit jam/jelly, apple "butter" (pureed apple), or pureed fresh fruit.

- Mix together, label, and store in refrigerator.

Calories:

3 calories per tablespoon, 65 calories per 1/2 cup (dessert)

Tips:
- A delicious lo-cal spread on pancakes, muffins, or toast.
- Eat plain as flavored yogurt for a tasty dessert—or an emergency meal. The yogurt provides easy calcium and protein in an otherwise all-carbohydrate meal.

OTHER YOGURT TRICKS

For vegetable dip or cracker spread, baked potato topping or skins, add one of the following to yogurt:
1. Salsa
2. Fresh or dried herbs of your choice. Experiment. For example, add chives and dried onions for potato topping.

DESSERTS/SNACKS

RANDY'S GO JUICE

(From Southwestern Bell's president, Randy Barron)
1 banana
1 cup orange juice
1 orange and/or grapefruit
1 carrot
1 apple
Strawberries—a "few"

1. Choose any combination and amounts of these ingredients.
2. Blend together in blender.

Tips:

- I take the liberty to suggest using frozen fruit or lots of ice and blend until ice is crushed. Blend in some pineapple juice for a cool summer Pina Colada-type drink.
- Randy drinks this for a quick pick up instead of soda.

PAULA KENT MEEHAN'S 5-MINUTE PIE

(Redken's CEO)

1 package Crokine Crackers (by General Biscuits)
2–4 cups fresh, frozen, or canned (unsweetened) fruit
sweetener (not sugar)

1. Spread crackers on bottom of pie tin.
2. Cover with fruit—for example—strawberries, blueberries, peaches.
3. Sprinkle with a safe sweetener such as Barleymalt Sweetener or fructose.

Bake:

350 degrees for 5 minutes

Calories:

Approximately 50 calories per slice

Tips:

- Crokine crackers are 19 calories each (General Biscuits) and are a light, puffed crispbread.
- Use comparable alternatives for Crokine if unavailable such as apple cinnamon Crispy Cakes (Pacific Rice Products, 20 calories each). Both are sold in regular grocery stores.

FROZEN NUTTY BANANAS

(A great, cool, summertime meal)

ripe bananas (when black flecks begin to appear on peel)
crushed peanuts, sunflower seeds (put in bag and use rolling pin or bottle)
oat bran

1. Peel bananas.
2. Put crushed mix in plastic bag.
3. Put banana in same bag and gently squeeze mix into banana from the outside of bag.

4. Put on cookie sheet and shove Popsicle stick (hobby store) into end of banana.
5. Put in freezer, uncovered, until frozen.
6. Wrap individually and store in freezer.

Calories:
150 each

Tips:
• This is a great snack or "emergency meal" in the summertime.
• Plain frozen bananas are also very tasty (without the peanuts).

FROZEN GRAPES

(Warning—this recipe is only for advanced cooks!)
1. Place unwashed, separated grapes in freezer (in plastic container or bag).
2. Rinse grapes just before eating.

Calories:
50 calories per 1/2 cup

FROZEN (OR UNFROZEN) YOGURT

32 oz. plain nonfat yogurt
1/3 teaspoon Barleymalt Sweetener (powdered)
2 drops flavoring—vanilla, strawberry, etc.

1. Mix and store in refrigerator or put in small serving dishes (champagne glasses are nice), top with strawberry or other fruit, sprinkle with oat bran, and freeze (carefully).
2. Take out at start of meal to let thaw a bit. Serve for dessert.

Calories:
35–50 per 1/3 cup (depending on yogurt)

NO
EXCUSES

Chapter Twelve

YOUR MENU PLANNING STRATEGY

MAKING THE RECIPES OF SPEED COOKING PART OF YOUR DAILY ROUTINE

Developing your wellness potential is simple economics.

—*Malcolm Stamper, Boeing Company*

Whether you have a family or are eating alone, you should make your meals an event. Use your best dishes, glasses, and silverware—or buy one or two fun settings. Stock up on candles too. It takes no extra time to make your meals aesthetically pleasing. If lighting a candle seems like too much trouble, consider the Japanese tea ceremony—two hours to make a cup of tea, and they still have time to be world industry leaders. Also, keep the television off. Put on some soft music and just taste the food. Put the fork down between bites and chew the food slowly, thoroughly, and in an undriven manner (see Motivation, Step #9, Scanning, page 104). When the meal is over, you will be less inclined to snack in the evening because your eating experience will have been complete, and you won't feel as though you have to make up for being deprived. In treating eating as an art, you will increase your awareness (and thus satisfaction) of every bite. Increased satisfaction means less mindless stuffing, fewer calories ingested, and a flatter stomach.

YOUR GUIDE TO WEEKLY MENU PLANNING

As discussed earlier, most people eat only about ten different meals. With that in mind, you can see that by mixing and matching ingredients and foods, you can build on your "Basic Ten" and add variety to your menu effortlessly.

Start with the following plan and you will soon get the hang of Speed Cooking in relation to your new menu strategy. You will learn that besides cooking individual recipes in large quantities for future use, it is also productive and surprisingly easy to cook several different recipes simultaneously. You can learn to work with the ingredients you have on hand and try new ideas as you go. Ideally, you can cook (and shop) just once a week (Sunday evening is ideal for many), creating your week's supply as well as building a sumptuous reserve.

Your menu will be varied and based on your tastes, but the following four-week sample menu will give you an idea of how it goes. Also included is a sample dinner menu for each week based on that week's cooking, as well as your reserve. "Graze" means having a *very* light dinner—yogurt, raw vegetables, fruit, popcorn, rice cakes, or salad (a good practice to break the "three hot squares" mentality). (Use the recipes described in Chapter 11.)

Week 1 Cooking

Chicken Pilaf   Chicken Soup

Chicken and Rice Picante   Rice

Chicken and Rice Curry   Multiway Salad

WEEK 1 DINNER SHOPPING LIST:

(Use HWW Shopping List)

red snapper
12–14 lbs. chicken
green onions
1 bunch carrots
1 bunch celery
Pace Picante Sauce (medium)
1 pkg. frozen peas
2 nonfat plain yogurt (32 oz. size)
2 pkgs. brown rice
lettuce
1 head purple cabbage

fruit
whole wheat rolls
sunflower seeds, sliced almonds or pine nuts
raisins
curry powder
tamari
Vege-Sal

Optional items:
1 pkg. low-fat cheese
mushrooms
salad additions—peppers, tomatoes, etc.

Tip:
Week 1 Cooking can be done in one session.

As the chicken is boiling, start the rice and then the salad. Many of the vegetables for the salad will also be used for the soup. You can either use this chicken broth for the soup or use a defatted broth from your freezer reserve. If you use this broth, go ahead and make the soup but don't eat it until it has cooled and you have skimmed off the fat. Boil a lot of chicken (12 to 14 pounds), because you will use it for the soup, the Chicken and Rice dishes and, if possible, have some left to freeze (on the bone or deboned or for sandwiches, Chinese dishes, snacks etc. Don't panic at the quantity—it will all be eaten, and you'll be grateful you planned ahead). Also, make a lot of rice (see Rice Recipes) for the Chicken and Rice dishes, Chicken Soup, and to store (plain, curry, Mexican, or Chinese rice). Label and freeze part of the rice, chicken, chicken soup, and *all* of the Chicken and Rice Picante and the Chicken and Rice Curry dishes. Leave enough of the Chicken and Rice Pilaf unfrozen for two meals. Leave enough of the Chicken Soup unfrozen for two meals.

WEEK 1 DINNER MENUS

Day	
1	Chicken and Rice Pilaf, salad, fruit
2	Red Snapper, salad, whole-wheat roll
3	Chicken Soup, salad, whole-wheat roll
4	Chicken and Rice Pilaf, salad, fruit
5	Chicken Soup, salad, whole-wheat roll
6	Rice Tostada, fruit
7	"Graze"

Note: "Day 1" is Sunday in this case. It is the day you shop and cook. Since it is wise to eat fish at least once a week and since it is best fresh, try to eat it on the day you shopped or the day after. The rolls are from your handy freezer stock. A full week is outlined to give you some ideas, although statistics show that most young business people dine out more than once a week. Leftovers can be eaten for lunch (soup and pilaf). "Grazing" has been previously described. (Be careful not to use this as an excuse to nibble your way to fatdom.)

Week 2 Cooking

Lentil Soup

Black Bean Soup

Hot Black Bean Soup

Multiway Soup

Yams

WEEK 2 DINNER SHOPPING LIST

(Use HWW Shopping List)

swordfish

2 pkgs. lentils

2 pkgs. black beans

2 red onions

yams (2–3 per person)

1 bunch carrots

lettuce

fruit

1 head purple cabbage

thyme

basil

whole-wheat rolls

salsa

salad optional additions

Tips:

Week 2 cooking can be done in one session.

The recipes for Lentil Soup and Black Bean Soup are essentially the same, so you simply get two (large) pots going at the same time. (Feel free to make one or two additional soups if you have the pans.) Either split the Black Bean Soup recipe (finished product) in half to make Hot Black Bean Soup with half or make a full recipe of the "hot" version. It takes little more effort. As before, some of the salad vegetables will be used in the soup. Make two to three yams per person. They are handy to have around for eating cold (or reheating) as dessert (add a touch of cinnamon), as a snack, or with a meal. You will freeze part of the Lentil Soup and most of the Black Bean Soups.

WEEK 2 DINNER MENUS

Day	
1	Swordfish, yam, salad
2	Lentil Soup, whole-wheat roll, salad, fruit
3	Black Bean Soup, yam (cold or reheated), fruit
4	Rice (freezer stock) with Lentil Dahl (see Soup Recipes), salad
5	Chicken and Rice Curry (freezer stock), fruit
6	Chicken and Rice Curry (leftover from day 5)
7	Potato Tostada or "graze"

Week 3 Cooking (Easy Week)

Pasta Primavera
Multiway Salad

WEEK 3 DINNER SHOPPING LIST:

(Use HWW Shopping List)
Dover sole
spiral whole wheat pasta
1 head broccoli
1 head cauliflower
1 red and/or yellow pepper
1 bunch carrots
frozen peas and/or corn
feta cheese
lettuce
1 head purple cabbage
salad optional additions
fruit

Tip:
Week three cooking can be done in one session.

• Freeze part of the Pasta Primavera, if leftovers are predicted.

WEEK 3 DINNER MENUS

Day	
1	Hot Pasta Primavera, Multiway Salad
2	Dover Sole, cold Pasta Primavera over Multiway Salad
3	Hot Black Bean Soup (freezer stock), whole-wheat roll, fruit
4	Cold Pasta Primavera over Multiway Salad, whole-wheat roll
5	Steamed Vegetables over rice (freezer stock), fruit
6	"Graze" or freezer recruit
7	Chicken Soup (freezer stock), whole-wheat roll, fruit

Week 4 Cooking—Recruit Week

Multiway Salad

WEEK 4 DINNER SHOPPING LIST: (OPTIONAL)

(Use HWW Shopping List)
halibut
baking potatoes
lettuce
1 head purple cabbage
1 bunch carrots
avocado
fruit
salad optional additions

    While it is better to do a little shopping on these Recruit Weeks (for fresh fruit, vegetables, fish), you *could* get by without shopping once in a while, if you've done your homework. It comes in handy with an especially busy work week.

WEEK 4 DINNER MENU

Day	
1	Poached halibut, baked potato, salad
2	Black Bean Dahl over rice (freezer stock), Multiway salad
3	Potato Tostada with avocado, fruit
4	Chicken and Rice Picante (freezer stock), fruit
5	"Graze" (fruit, popcorn)
6	Chicken and Rice Picante
7	Lentil Soup (freezer stock), whole-wheat roll, fruit

A SAMPLE WEEKLY MENU

The following menu should give you an overview of how a given week might look using the recipes and ideas in this book—breakfast, lunch, and dinner. The selections are simple, nutritious, and delicious.

Day	Breakfast	Lunch	Dinner
Monday	Shepherd's Granola	Chicken Sandwich	Red Snapper
Tuesday	Oatmeal	Tuna Salad	Chicken and Broccoli
Wednesday	Muffin	Veggie Sandwich	Tostada
Thursday	Cottage Cheese on Toast	Pasta Salad	Poached Salmon
Friday	Shepherd's Granola	Vegetable Soup	Potato Tostada
Saturday	Pancakes	Tuna Sandwich	Dahl with rice
Sunday	Poached Eggs	Graze	Chinese food

EMERGENCY EATERY TIPS

If you are behind on your weekly freezer-stocking, or you are feeling lazy, it's nice to have a few trustworthy cans of healthful food in the cupboard. All you need is a well-stocked kitchen. Following are some ideas to see you through emergencies—and you can get more ideas by browsing through your health-food store. Buying at a good health-food store usually ensures higher-quality ingredients and more healthful choices, but check the labels.

(1) Can or jar: vegetarian chili, pilaf, amaranth or lentil hot-dishes (Health Valley has some good choices), vegetarian spaghetti sauce, etc.

(2) Frozen: vegeburgers, chicken or turkey hot dogs (watch sodium), frozen dinners

(3) Boxed: tabouli (great in pita bread), hummus

If you are too busy to take a lunch break, please try to eat *something*. This will eliminate ulcers, low energy, and the tendency to binge later in the day. Following are items that are semi-nonperishable so that you can actually "stock" your desk, car or briefcase as part of your (weekly) routine. If not, you can easily pick up most of them at a nearby convenience store (versus grabbing the wrong thing when you're in a hurry or when you haven't thought it out). You may not think of these items as "meals", but they will do in a pinch.

1. Rice cakes
2. Bran muffins (watch out for sugar and oil—make your own)
3. Fruit (especially apples—long shelf life and unsquishable)
4. Raw almonds
5. Trail mix (make your own—raw and unsalted)

Eight Great Breakfast Ideas

Most of the menu planning concerns dinner, since lunch is often eaten out. It's a good idea to have a rotating repertoire of breakfast ideas as well, since you should always look forward to, and enjoy, each meal. Besides, ruts can cause a sensitivity (allergy) to a food if it is eaten day after day. Sometimes we forget a good idea and get dull, so it's useful to keep a list of ideas for future reference. Incidentally, eat fruit on an empty stomach, if possible, and eat at least ten minutes before any other food to aid the digestive process.

Here are some nutritious and delicious breakfast ideas:

1. Oatmeal—instant packets (Erewhon is a good nonsugar brand, 130 calories), or homemade steelcut (sold in packages or bulk) is deliciously grainy and chewy and can be reheated for two to three days. Add "cinnamon sugar" (cinnamon sweetened with fructose or Barleymalt Sweetener), dates, raisins, or almonds. Cooked steelcut oatmeal is even good cold as a quick snack.
2. Bran muffins—preferably homemade with no oil and no sugar (see recipes).
3. Yogurt—self sweetened or unsweetened (See Chapter 4, Breakfast Tips).
4. Toast with: all-fruit jams, cottage cheese, 1/4 avocado, tofu (mix tofu with "cinnamon sugar" until smooth and spread on lightly toasted bread, then sprinkle with "cinnamon sugar" and bake in toaster oven on low at 250 degrees for five to ten minutes. Delicious!)
5. HWW Shepherd's Granola—homemade raw granola (see recipes).
6. Store-bought cereals—more acceptable ones are popping up daily. Acceptable old nutritious standbys: Grapenuts, Shredded Wheat, Nutri-Grain. Check labels for sugar, fats, and preservatives.

7. Egg white omelette or scrambled (use all egg whites or one whole egg and two to three egg whites). Add onions, green/red/yellow peppers, low-fat cheese, mushrooms or herbs.

8. Pancakes, waffles—use healthful mixes (Hain's is great). Use all-fruit spread, apple butter, HWW Fruit Spread, or cinnamon sugar (see #1) instead of syrup and butter. Use two egg whites for every egg suggested and Yogurt Milk or nonfat milk instead of whole milk—cuts down fat and calories.

Your additions:

9.

10.

11.

12.

13.

14.

STOCKING YOUR KITCHEN SUCCESSFULLY

The best plan hasn't got a chance unless you are building on a solid foundation. In this case, you need a properly stocked kitchen. Don't worry—this is a surprisingly simple and basic setup. It will probably mean one quick trip to one store to get the job done (and remember, someone else can do this for you, if you can arrange it).

Handy Utensils to Have on Hand

(Circle those you need to purchase)

1. Large saucepans—12"–14", nonstick
2. Small saucepans—6"–8", nonstick
3. Soup pots—6–12 quart size, not aluminum

4. Casserole pans—8″ × 8″ to 12″ × 16″, depending on family size (oven and freezer proof)
5. Blender
6. Steamer—double decker, not aluminum
7. Freezer bags and/or various size plastic containers for freezing and one container for a large "week's worth" salad (6–8 quart size)

Optional:

8. Muffin tins
9. Food processor
10. Pressure cooker (cooks beans much faster)
11. A large freezer . . .

Food in the Freezer Is Like Money in the Bank: How to Stock Your Freezer

1. Rice
2. Beans
3. Soups
4. Breads, rolls, pita bread, muffins, tortillas, buns (all whole wheat)
5. Vegetables (certain ones, such as peas, corn, lima beans)
6. Vegeburgers, tofu, chicken, or turkey hot dogs
7. Casseroles and other homemade meals—family and individual sizes
8. Chicken Stock
9. Chicken—cooked (cut up or on the bone) and/or uncooked

Your additions:

10.

11.

12.

13.

14.

How to Stock Your Cupboards

The following items should be added to your cupboards:

1. Rice cakes
2. Refried beans
3. Sweetener—powdered barleymalt or fructose; canned, unsweetened, crushed pineapple
4. Dried beans, peas, lentils, rice
5. Mexican salsa, spaghetti sauce
6. Pasta—whole grain (different types for various dishes)
7. Extra dressing (keep a lot on hand)
8. Canned meals (from health-food store)—amaranth pilaf (wheat free), chili, tuna
9. Herbs: Vege-Sal (or other salt flavoring), basil, garlic powder, onion powder, tabasco, cayenne, curry powder, cinnamon, oregano, and vanilla.

Your additions:

10.

11.

12.

13.

14.

How to Stock Your Refrigerator

1. Liquid Aminos (or soy-sauce flavoring)—health-food store
2. Quick Sip (or other nonsalt, all-purpose flavoring—soup stocks etc.)
3. Tamari
4. Dijon mustard
5. Salad dressings
6. Plain nonfat yogurt
7. Fruit—put in basket on top shelf (visible and pretty)
8. Oils—preferably canola or olive oil or ghee (purified butter)

9. "Mayo" (see recipes)

10. Low-fat cheese, regular and Parmesan type (dried and grated)

11. Vegetables—potatoes, yams, broccoli, lettuce

12. All-fruit jam, apple butter

Your Additions:

13.

14.

15.

16.

17.

THE ULTIMATE SHOPPING LIST

The following list is a useful tool to help ensure that you always have everything you need on hand. It can also help you avoid countless one-item trips to the grocery store. The list is divided between two basic stores: a regular grocery store and a health-food store. The idea is that you make one trip to one or both stores once a week only. In fact, many of my single clients buy most of their weekly supplies at the health-food store and have simplified their regular grocery store trips to once every three or four weeks (just to buy stock items such as paper products and sparkling water). Always buy the best-tasting, best-quality food you can—you're worth it. You may photocopy The Ultimate Shopping List for your own individual use.

Recommended Products:

1. Barleymalt Sweetener
   By: Bronner, Escondido, CA

2. Vege-Sal (Gayelord Hauser)
   By: Modern Products, Milwaukee, WI

3. Ghee (purified butter)
   By: Purity Farms, Silver Spring, MD

4. Liquid Aminos
   By: Live Food Products, Santa Barbara, CA

5. Quick Sip
   By: Bernard Jensen, Solana Beach, CA
6. Lifetime Cheese
   By: Lifeline Food Co., Seaside, CA
   or
   Vitalait Cheese
   By: Cabot Farmer's Cooperative, Cabot, VT
7. Chili
   By: Health Valley, Irwindale, CA
   (This company has a wonderful line of foods—all delicious.)
8. Whole Wheat Baking Mix
   By: Hain Pure Food Co., Los Angeles, CA

THE ULTIMATE SHOPPING LIST

REGULAR GROCERY STORE:

PROTEIN
Fish ___
Chicken ___
Turkey ___
Other ___
___

GRAINS
Bread ___
Rolls/buns ___
Muffins ___
Rice ___
Pasta ___
Oatmeal ___
Cereal ___
Dried beans ___
Other ___
___

DAIRY
Milk ___
Yogurt ___
Cheese ___
Other ___
___

PRODUCE
Fruit ___
___
___
___
Vegetables ___
Lettuce ___
Carrots ___
Tomatoes ___
Broccoli ___
Other ___
___

FROZEN FOODS
___
___
___
___

CANNED FOODS
___
___
___
___

SNACKS
Popcorn ___
Other ___
___

BEVERAGES
___
___
___

MISCELLANEOUS
Toothpaste ___
Shampoo ___
Other ___
___

HERBS, CONDIMENTS, SALAD DRESSING, etc.
Mustard ___
Salad Dressing ___
___
Lemon juice ___
Vanilla, etc. ___
Oil ___
Herbs ___
Other ___
___

CLEANING/GENERAL
Paper towels ___
Toilet tissue ___
Tissues ___
Napkins ___
Alum. foil ___
Plastic wrap ___
Plastic bags ___
Cleaning supplies ___
___
Light bulbs ___
Other ___

HEALTH-FOOD STORE:

VITAMINS
_____
_____

PROTEIN
Fish _____
Chicken _____
Turkey _____
Other _____

GRAINS
Bread _____
Roll/buns _____
Muffins _____
Rice _____
Pasta _____
Oatmeal _____
Cereal _____
Dried beans _____
Other _____
_____
_____
_____
_____

PRODUCE
Fruit _____
_____
_____
Vegetables _____
_____
_____

DAIRY
Yogurt _____
Cheese _____
Milk _____
Other _____
_____
_____
_____
_____
_____
_____
_____

CANNED
Beans _____
Soups _____
Salsa _____
Tuna _____
Other _____

FROZEN
Dinners _____
Veggies _____
Other _____

BEVERAGES
_____
_____
_____
_____
_____

HERBS, CONDIMENTS
SALAD DRESSINGS
Herbs _____
_____
Sweeteners _____
Oils _____
Jams _____
Vanilla, etc. _____
Stocks _____
Mustard _____
Other _____

SNACKS
_____
_____

MISCELLANEOUS
_____
_____
_____
_____
_____

271

*B*IBLIOGRAPHY

Abraham, S., Johnson, C.L., and Carrol, M.D. Total serum cholesterol level of adults 18–74 years of age: United States, 1971–74. Report prepared for *Advance Data*, Vital & Health Statistics, U.S. Dept. of HEW, May 25, 1977, 7, 1–7.

American Cancer Society. Cancer facts and figures. 1985.

American Health. March 1985, 126; October 1986; March 1987; April 1987; May 1987; November 1987; December 1987, 22, 42, 58, 89; January 1988, 43; March 1988; April 1988; May 1988; September 1988; November 1988; December 1988; March 1989, 46; April 1989; May 1989, 22; October 1990.

American Journal of Psychiatry. October 1974.

APFC Newsletter. Rodale Press, October/November 1984.

Ballentine, R., M.D. *Diet & Nutrition*, 1978, 557–559.

Banister, E.W. Health, Fitness and Productivity, *Labour Gazette*, Canada, September 1978, 78(9), 400–407.

Barrie, K., et al. Mental distress as a problem for industry. *Mental Wellness Programs for Employees*, eds. Richard H. Egdahl and Diana C. Walsh, n.d.

Beehr, T.A. and Newman, J.E. Job stress, employee health, and organizational effectiveness: A facet analysis, model, and literature review. *Personal Psychology*, 1978, 31(4), 665–699.

Beehr, T.A., Walsh, J.T., and Tabor, T.D. Relationships of stress to individually and organizationally valued states: Higher order needs as a moderator. *Journal of Applied Psychology*, 1976, 61(1), 41–47.

Bellows, E.H. and Gasque, M.R. Here's a lifesaving plan for your business. *Nation's Business*, April 1966, 94.

Bennett, William and Gurin, J. *The Dieter's Dilemma*. 1982

Bernacki, E.J. and Baun, W.B. The relationship of job performance to exercise adherence in a corporate fitness program. *Journal of Occupational Medicine*, July 1984, 26(7), 529–531.

Berry, C.A. *Good Health for Employees and Reduced Health Care Costs for Industry*. Health insurance Association of America, 1981.

Bogert, J., Briggs, G., and Calloway, D. *Nutrition and Physical Fitness*. Pennsylvania: W.B. Saunders Co., 1973.

Buscaglia, L. *Living, Loving & Learning*. New York: Ballantine Books, 1982.

Business Week. The executive under pressure, May 25, 1974.

Carroll, V. Employee fitness program: An expanding concept. *International Journal of Health Education*, 1981, 26, 35–41.

Castelli, W.P., M.D. Categorical issues in therapy for coronary heart disease. *Cardiology in Practice*, January/February 1985, 267–73.

Reversing the course of atherosclerosis—A view from Framingham. *Current Concepts*, April 1989, 32–36.

Cherry, N. Stress, anxiety and work: A longitudinal study. *Journal of Occupational Psychology*, 1978, 51(3), 259–270.

Colligan, M.J., Smith, M.J., and Hurrell, J.J. Occupational incidence rates of mental disorders. *Journal of Human Stress*, 1977, 3(3), 34–39.

Conway, T.L., et al. Occupational stress and variation in cigarette, coffee and alcohol consumption. *Journal of Health & Social Behavior*, 1981, 22(2), 155–165.

Cooper, C.L. and Marshall, J. Occupational sources of stress: A review of the literature relating to coronary heart disease and mental ill health. *Occupational Psychology*, 1976, 49(1), 11–28.

Cooper, C.L. and Melhuish, A. Executive stress and health. *Journal of Occupational Medicine*, February 1984, 26(2), 99–104.

Chronobiologica. 1976, 3(1).

Cummings, L.L. and Decotiis, T.A. Organizational correlates of perceived stress in a professional organization. *Public Personnel Management*, 1973, 2(4), 275–282.

Danchik, K.M., Schoenborn, C.A., and Elinson, J. Highlights from wave I of the national survey of personal health practices and consequences: United States, 1979. Report prepared for Vital & Health Statistics of the National Center for Health Statistics, U.S. Dept. of the HEW, June 1981, 15(1), 1–24.

de Bono, E. *Tactics: The Art and Science of Success*. Boston: Little, Brown, & Co., 1984.

Dept. of Agriculture. Maintain ideal weight. *Nutrition and Your Health,* U. S. Dept. of Health & Human Services, February, 1980, 8. Cited from HEW conference on obesity, 1973.

Dishman, R.K., editor. *Exercise Adherence: Its Impact on Public Health,* 1988.

Donohue, S. The correlation between physical fitness, absenteeism, and work performance. *Canadian Journal of Public Health,* 1977, 68, 201–203.

Dun & Bradstreet. *Dun's Business Rankings, 1984,* 1019–1021.

Dun's Business Month. Executive health audit: Special report, October 1984, 88–112.

Eisenstadt, R.K. and Schoenborn, C.A. Basic data form wave II of the national survey of personal health practices and consequences: United States, 1980. *Working Paper Series.* Report prepared for the Office of Analysis and Epidemiology Program, U.S. Dept. of HEW, October 1982, 13, 8–20.

Emerson, J. Cholesterol: The most misunderstood nutrient. *Whole Life Times,* November/December 1984, 21–26.

Employee Physical Fitness in Canada: Proceedings of the National Conference on Employee Physical Fitness, 1975, 33.

Executive Edge, Vol. 21, August 1990.

Family Economics Review. Nutritive value of food intakes: Results from the USDA nationwide food consumption survey 1977–78, Summer 1981. Cited by Vitamin Nutrition Information Service, *VNIS Nutri-Stats,* 1984, RCD 3934-1–RCD 3934-3.

Financial Enterprise. Spring 1988.

Food & Nutrition, October 1990; December 1990.

Forbes. July 25, 1988.

Friedman, M. and Ulmer, D. *Treating Type A Behavior and Your Heart.* New York: Knopf, 1984.

Gallo, R.E. and Blaylock, J.R. Foods not eaten by Americans. *National Food Review–15,* USDA Economic Research Service, Summer 1981, 24, cited by Vitamin Nutrition Information Service, *VNIS Nutri-Stats,* 1984, RCD 4355-1–RCD 4355-4.

Gallup Organization. *Gallup Study of Vitamin Use in the United States.* Survey 6, vol. 1, Princeton, N.J., 1982, cited by Vitamin Nutrition Information Service, *VNIS Nutri-Stats,* 1984, RCD 3976-1–RCD 3976-2.

Garn, S.M. Socioeconomic aspects of obesity. *Contemporary Nutrition,* 1981, 6(7).

Glomset, J.A. Fish, fatty acids and human health. *New England Journal of Medicine,* 1985, 312(19), 1253.

Goldbeck, W.B. Psychiatry and industry: A business view. *The Psychiatric Hospital,* 1982, 13(3) 95–98.

Greiff, B.S. and Munster, P.K. *Tradeoffs—Executive Family and Organizational Life.* New York: New American Library, 1980.

Harris, T.G. and Gurin, J. Look who's getting it all together. *American Health,* March 1985, 42–47.

Health Insurance Association of America. For controlling employee health care costs. *Time* magazine special advertising section, June 18, 1984.

Health News Digest. December 1987.

Hoffman, J.J. and Hobson, C.J. Physical fitness and employee effectiveness. *Personnel Administrator*, April 1984, 101–113.

Industry Week. Executive—healthy but out of shape, 14 October, 1974, 183(2), 50–58.

International Lipid Information Bureau. April 1988.

Jobin, J. The new type-E woman. *Self*, January 1985, 56–57.

Johnson, H.J. *Executive Life Styles: A Life Extension Institute Report on Alcohol, Sex, & Health*. New York: T.Y. Crowell Co., 1974.

Jonas, S. and Silver, N. The last cure-all. *American Health*, March 1985, 63–64.

Journal of the American Medical Association. April 15,1988; July 1, 1982; August 7, 1981.

Journal of Applied Nutrition. 33(1), 1981.

Journal of Occupational Medicine. November 1984, 26(11).

Kaufman, J.E. State of the art: Physical fitness in corporations. *Employee Services Management*, February 1983, 8.

Keenan, A. and Mc Bain, G.D. Effect of Type A behavior, intolerance of ambiguity, and locus of control on the relationship between role stress and work-related outcomes. *Journal of Occupational Psychology*, 1979, 52(4), 277–285.

Kopbasa, S.C. Personality and resistance to illness. *American Journal of Community Psychology*, 1979, 7(4), 413–423.

Kromhout, D., Bosschieter, E., and Coulander, C. The inverse relationship between fish consumption and 20-year mortality from coronary heart disease. *New England Journal of Medicine*, 1985, 312(19), 1205–7.

Kundalini Yoga Sadhana Guidelines, 1978, 30.

Levinson, H. Power, leadership, and the management of stress. *Professional Psychology*, 1980, 11(3), 497–508.

———*Executive Stress*. New York: New American Library, revised and updated, 1975.

Los Angeles Times. Exercise! Workouts fight depression and increase esteem. Special advertising supplement, 11 April 1985, pt. 5, 30. Also April 29, 1990, pt.2.

Lynch, J.J. Listen and live. *American Health*, April 1985, 39–43.

Louis Harris & Associates, Inc. *The Prevention Index: A Report Card on the Nation's Health*. Commissioned by *Prevention* magazine, 1983.

———*The Perrier Study: Fitness in America*. New York: Perrier, 1979.

Margolis, B. and Kroes, W. Work and the health of man. *Work and the Quality of Life*, O'Toole J., Cambridge, Mass.: MIT Press, 1974.

Market Research Corporation of America Information Services. Americans' snacking habits analyzed. *Better Nutrition*, July 1985, 45(7), 7–8.

Matousek, O. and Hladky, A. Man and the stress aspect of work. *Synteza*, 1971, 4(5), 137–144.

Mayo Clinic Nutrition Letter. December 1988, 1(9); February 1990.

Medical Tribune. FP headache rate high. June 10, 1981, 22, 17.

Metropolitan Life Insurance Company, *1983 Metropolitan Height and Weight Tables*, Health and Safety Education Division, 1983.

McCall, M.W. and Lombardo, M.M. What makes a top executive? *Best of Business*, 1983, 5(2), 82–86.

Mirkin, G. and Hoffman, M. *The Sportsmedicine Book.* Boston: Little, Brown & Co., 1978.

Mirkin, G. *Getting Thin.* Boston: Little, Brown & Co., 1983.

Mlachack, N.N. Glamour and junkets—or heroic patience? *Industry Week*, October 1984, 75–80.

National Health Survey, Respondent-assessed health status by selected characteristics. *Americans Assess their Health: United States, 1978*, U.S. Dept. of Health & Human Services, March 1983, 10(142), 7–17.

Natural Health and Fitness Bulletin. January 1987.

New England Journal of Medicine. December 16, 1982.

Newsweek. The losing formula. April 30, 1990, 52.

Nutrition Action Healthletter. January/February 1989, published by the Center for Science in the Public Interest, November 1990.

Oliver, P.L. and Kirkpatrick, M. Employee health enhancement: A new corporate challenge. *Health Care Industry Service*, Arthur D. Little Decision Resources, March 1982, 1–8.

Pauly J.T., Palmer, J.A., and Wright, C.C. The effects of a 14-week employee fitness program on selected psychological parameters. *Journal of Occupational Medicine*, 1982, 24, 457–62.

Perry, P. Dawn on the fast track. *American Health*, March 1985, 48–51.

Phillips, A.M. A study of prolonged absenteeism in industry. *Journal of Occupational Medicine*, 1961.

Plateris, A.A. Duration of marriage before divorce: United States. National Center for Health Statistics, U.S. Dept. of Health & Human Services, Public Health Service, July 1981, 21(38), 1–13.

President's Council on Physical Fitness and Sports. Employee fitness: Corporate philosophy for the 1980's. *Athletic Purchasing and Facilities.* July 1980, 12–14.

Prevention. June 1983, 69–73; April 1983, 59.

Reuben, C. Gut issues: Fat is to the intestine what cigarette smoke is to the lungs. *L.A. Weekly*, August 1985, R–7.

Reynolds, R. Corporate fitness means good business. *Research Institute*, Cooper Clinic, June 1983, 4(4), 1.

Richman, L.S. Health benefits come under the knife. *Fortune*, May 2, 1983, 95–110.

Roberts, J. and Maurer, K. Blood pressure of persons 6–74 years of age in the United States. Report prepared for *Advance Data*, Vital and Health Statistics, U.S. Dept. of HEW, October 18, 1976, 1, 1–6.

Roark, A.C. Are We as Fit as We Think? *Los Angeles Times Good Health Magazine*, 15, 30.

Ruch, R. and Goodman, R. Image at the top. *Best of Business*, 1983, 5(2), 44–53.

Runner's World. April, 1988, 69.

Sarason, I.G. and Johnson, J.H. Life, stress, organizational stress, and job satisfaction. *Psychological Reports*, 1979, 44(10), 305–317.

Schoenborn, C. A. and Danchik, K.M. Educational differentials in health practices. *Health United States*, Public Health Services, U.S. Dept. of HEW, 1981, 33–38.

Scientific American. Diet and cancer. November 1987, 257(5).

SmithKline Bio-Science Laboratories, *Service Manual*, May 1, 1985, 53, 119.

Statistical Bulletin. Longevity of corporate executives. February 1974.

Stix, H. Stress and working people: New program in Oakland. *Los Angeles Times*, September 11,1984, pt. 5, 1, 5.

Syme, S.L. and Berkman, L.F. Social class, susceptibility, and sickness. *American Journal of Epidemiology*, 1976, 104, 1–8.

Tennis Magazine, Health and Fitness Guide. May 1988.

Trost Associates, Inc. *Executive Summary: Benchmark National Study*. Prepared for Hoffman-La Roche Inc., April 1981, 1–16.

Tufts University Diet and Nutrition Letter. Vol 8, No. 5, July 1990; Vol 8, No. 7, September 1990; Vol 8, No. 12, February 1991.

University of California, Berkeley Wellness Letter, December 1989, February 1990, March 1990, October 1990; Vol 7, No. 12, September 1991.

U.S. Health Inc. Profile developed on spa members, Cited in the *APFC Newsletter*, October/November 1984, 5.

Villa Dresser, C.M., Carroll, M.D., and Abraham, S. Selected findings: Food consumption profiles of white and black persons 1–74 years of age in the United States, 1971–74. Report prepared for *Advance Data*, Vital & Health Statistics, U.S. Dept. of HEW, June 26, 1978, 21, 1–7.

Wachta, P.H. Exercising prerogatives. *Management Focus*, Peat Marwick, November, 1984, 30–35.

Walford, R.L., M.D. *Maximum Life Span*, 1983.

Walking Magazine. March 1988, 40.

Wallach, Leah. *Food Values: Cholesterol & Fats*, 1989.

Washington Business Group on Health. Worksite health evaluation report. *Corporate Commentary*, November 1984, (2), 1–71.

Wilder, C.S. Disability days: United States, 1980. National Center for Health Statistics, U.S. Dept. of Health & Human Services, Public Health Service, July 1983, 10(143), 22–23; and Selected health characteristics by occupation: United States 1975–76. National Center for Health Statistics, U.S. Dept. of Health and Human Services, May, 1980, 10(133), 1–2.

Williams, P. Stanford Center for Research & Disease Prevention, Stanford, CA. Interview, June 6, 1985.

Williams, P., et al. Coffee intake and elevated cholesterol and apolipo-protein B levels in men. *Journal of the American Medical Association*, March 8, 1985, 253(10), 1407–1411.

Wright, P. The harassed decision maker: Time pressures, distractions and the use of evidence. *Journal of Applied Psychology*, 1974, 59(5), 555–561.

Yankelovitch, Skelly & White, Inc. *Monitor*, 1978–1980. Cited by Vitamin Nutrition Information Service, *VNIS Nutri-Stats*, 1984, RCD 3714-1.

Your Personal Best. Vol 2, No. 9, September 1990.

INDEX

KRS' Tools for Self-Improvement

1. Healthy, Wealthy & Wise

"An entertaining book that has it all—a unique collection of motivation strategies with a 'failure-proof' diet/exercise/stress program that yields success in mind, body and life. Turns a busy lifestyle into a productive and balanced HealthStyle."
- Shirley Koster, wife, mother, M.S., R.D., Tucson Medical Center

2. Conquering Stress

A succinct, "get results" guidebook that takes you from "coping" with stress to conquering it. Includes psychological and meditation techniques along with practical skills.

3. Inner Mastery Series

"Outstanding series! KRS' grounding voice woven with glorious music creates a wonderfully transformational journey within."
- White Swan Music

Guided meditation tapes that provide new solutions to old problems. KRS blends her own techniques from over 20 years experience together with age-old ones that not only deliver immediate results, but also impart new skills to draw on for a lifetime. Background music composed to facilitate your progress. Each audio tape 40 minutes. Played by United Airlines.

4. Time Out For Time In - NEW!

This thoughtful little "picture booklet" offers inviting ideas on making time for quality moments. In a simple but inspiring way, it shows how you can experience each moment to its fullest and how, in cultivating internal serenity, the external world becomes softer.

5. T-Shirt - "KRS Edstrom's Weekend Spa Retreat – Time Out For Time In"

If you haven't had the opportunity to attend KRS' special transformational retreats, this white cotton tee with tropically colored meditator-on-an-island-with-palm-tree design will make you *feel* like you have!

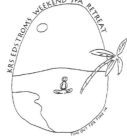

(order form on next page)

KRS' Tools for Self-Improvement
ORDER FORM

Item:	Price:	Quantity: (each)	Total Price:
1. *Healthy, Wealthy & Wise* (book)	$18.00	_____	_____
2. *Conquering Stress* (book)	$ 6.50	_____	_____
3. *Inner Mastery Series* (audio tapes)			
"Relax Mind & Body"	$12.00	_____	_____
"Defeat Pain"	$12.00	_____	_____
"Conquer Stress"	$12.00	_____	_____
"Sleep Through Insomnia"	$12.00	_____	_____
"Everyday Meditation"	$12.00	_____	_____
"Instrumentals I"	$12.00	_____	_____
6 Tape Series	$59.00	_____	_____
4. *Time Out For Time In* (booklet)	$ 6.50	_____	_____
5. "Time Out for Time In" T-shirt (Circle size: S M L XL)	$21.00	_____	_____

GRAND TOTAL enclosed:_____

SHIP TO:

Name _____

Address _____

City_____ State _____Zip_____

Phone *(optional)*_____

❏ Please keep me updated on KRS' retreats, lectures and new products

❏ I am interested in private phone sessions with KRS. Please call me.

Prices represent your total cost.

Send check payable to:

> **KRS**
> P.O. Box 8584
> Universal City, CA 91618-8584

Credit Card Orders for Tapes only: 1-800-888-4741
Credit Card Orders for *Healthy, Wealthy & Wise* only: 1-800-748-5804
Credit Card Orders for *Conquering Stress* book only: 1-800-645-3476

KRS' Tools for Self-Improvement
ORDER FORM

Item:	Price:	Quantity: (each)	Total Price:
1. *Healthy, Wealthy & Wise* (book)	$18.00	————	————
2. *Conquering Stress* (book)	$ 6.50	————	————
3. *Inner Mastery Series* (audio tapes)			
"Relax Mind & Body"	$12.00	————	————
"Defeat Pain"	$12.00	————	————
"Conquer Stress"	$12.00	————	————
"Sleep Through Insomnia"	$12.00	————	————
"Everyday Meditation"	$12.00	————	————
"Instrumentals I"	$12.00	————	————
6 Tape Series	$59.00	————	————
4. *Time Out For Time In* (booklet)	$ 6.50	————	————
5. "Time Out for Time In" T-shirt	$21.00	————	————

(Circle size: S   M   L   XL)

GRAND TOTAL enclosed:————

SHIP TO:

Name ————————————————————

Address ————————————————————

City———————————————— State ——— Zip————

Phone *(optional)* ————————————————

❏ Please keep me updated on KRS' retreats, lectures and new products

❏ I am interested in private phone sessions with KRS. Please call me.

Prices represent your total cost.
Send check payable to:

> **KRS**
> P.O. Box 8584
> Universal City, CA 91618-8584

Credit Card Orders for Tapes only: 1-800-888-4741
Credit Card Orders for *Healthy, Wealthy & Wise* only: 1-800-748-5804
Credit Card Orders for *Conquering Stress* book only: 1-800-645-3476